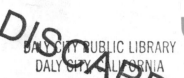

HEART FRAUDS

Uncovering the Biggest Health Scam in History

Charles T. McGee, M.D.

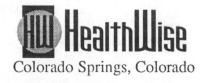
HealthWise
Colorado Springs, Colorado

W

Also by Charles T. McGee, M.D.
How to Survive Modern Technology
Miracle Healing From China...Qigong
Healing Energies

Published by **HealthWise Publications** an imprint of:
Piccadilly Books, Ltd.
P.O. Box 25203
Colorado Springs, CO 80936, USA

International sales and inquires contact:
 Empire Publishing Service
 20 Park Drive
 Romford Essex RM1 4LH, UK
or
 Empire Publishing Service
 P.O. Box 1344
 Studio City, CA 91614, USA

Library of Congress Cataloging-in-Publication Data
McGee, Charles T., 1935-
    Heart Frauds: uncovering the biggest health scam in history / Charles
    T. McGee.
       p. cm.
    Includes bibliographical references and index.
    ISBN 0-941599-56-6 (pbk.)
    1. Coronary heart disease--Etiology. 2. Medical misconceptions.
    3. Coronary heart disease--Treatment. 4. Hypercholesteremia.
    5. Transluminal angioplasty. 6. Coronary artery bypass. I. Title.
    RC685.C6 M365 2000
    616.1'23--dc21   00-025780

Simultaneously Published in Australia, UK, and USA
Printed in U.S.A.

TABLE OF CONTENTS

Thanks to:

My wife Carole for putting up with my pipe dreams.

David Pyle for his outrageous political cartoons.

Physicians who are able to adapt to new findings and change their beliefs and actions.

The late Robert Mendelsohn, M.D. who exposed so called "scientific medicine" as a religious belief system complete with infallible high priests (medical school professors), a canonized dogma, and an Inquisition reserved for heretics.

Dean Ornish, M.D., the first physician to prove beyond a shadow of a doubt that coronary artery disease can be reversed in the majority of people, and best of all, without drugs and surgery.

The late T.L. Cleave, British epidemiologist, who discovered why humans develop a long list of conditions known as diseases of physical degeneration.

Martha Zirschky and Vern Overlee for their special help in preparation of the manuscript.

Members of the American College of Advancement in Medicine for their support of innovation and progress in medicine.

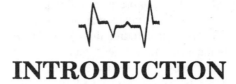

INTRODUCTION

Every year over 500,000 Americans die of coronary artery disease. Medicine has responded to this problem with a variety of preventive and treatment approaches. Some help, but the most common are very expensive, glamorized methods that do far *less* than most people are led to believe.

In the area of prevention, physicians recommend dietary measures based on the cholesterol theory. It may come as a surprise to you, but even after 40 years of relentless and expensive studies researchers have failed to prove the validity of the cholesterol theory. The fact is, blood cholesterol is only weakly associated with heart disease and between 1945 and 1995 not a single study presented evidence that reducing cholesterol blood levels would lower overall death rate. Some studies even showed that cholesterol-lowering drugs *increased* the overall death rate! Finally, in 1995 a study of one class of cholesterol-lowering drugs (statins) showed a decrease in heart attack death rate (but was as not effective as vitamin E as demonstrated in at least two studies). Zocor (a statin drug) soon was featured in television ads claiming to be the *first* cholesterol drug that actually did any good. Vitamin E which is far cheaper and safer is still generally ignored by the medical profession as a treatment for heart disease.

When symptoms of heart disease suddenly strike, patients are rushed to coronary care units of hospitals; the emergency response to life-threatening complications of heart attacks has saved many lives. In addition, many people also have made positive changes in their diets and lifestyles. The combination of these two has brought the annual death rate in people with known coronary artery disease down to under 2 percent, a level that can *not* be reduced any further with bypass surgeries or balloon angioplasties. Nonetheless, heart patients continue to be herded into these questionable and expensive procedures like sheep.

There are more problems. The ordinary angiogram used to *sell* bypasses and balloon procedures has been shown to be highly inaccurate. An accurate angiogram method was developed in the 1970s, but you and I can't get one. Its very existence has been treated almost like an insider's trade secret.

In the area of the angiogram, coronary artery bypass surgery, and balloon angioplasty, a pattern has been established. The procedures were developed and widely used before studies were completed that confirmed that they were either inaccurate of little value. When evidence appeared showing they were of little benefit, physicians simply chose to ignore it even though the articles were published in medical journals. Therefore, it is not surprising to learn that a second opinion clinic run by Harvard cardiologists found that over *80 percent* of bypasses and angiograms being recommended are not necessary.

The result is we are paying a high price in unnecessary pain and suffering as well as an estimated $45 billion in wasted health care expenditures per year. At a time when the cost of health care is threatening to bankrupt the nation we need to become aware of questionable practices within medicine that deserve to be modified or stopped entirely.

On the brighter side, it has been shown that coronary artery disease can be reversed without drugs or surgery. This information, combined with the new oxidation theory of the cause of atherosclerosis, leads directly to prevention and treatment approaches that *do* work and are far less expense and much more humane. However, these discoveries are not taught to physicians because vested interests in the medical/pharmaceutical/industrial complex resist changes that would hurt their profits.

If you had the choice between a safe, inexpensive, non-invasive procedure or a very costly method of treatment accompanied by the risk of dangerous side effects, which would you choose? In addition, what if your chances of success with the first procedure was far greater than the second? I think there is no question that you would choose the first. Unfortunately, you are rarely given a choice. The latter treatment, the one that is more expensive, carries greater health risks, and is less effective is the one prescribed by most doctors. In this book you will discover that you do have choices and you will learn what those choices are. With this knowledge you can avoid much of the pain and suffering that accompanies medical treatments. You will learn about and be able to recognize the *fraud* that exists in the health care industry as it applies to the treatment of heart disease. Webster's Dictionary defines "fraud" as deceit, trickery, and cheating. Fraud may seem like a harsh word to apply to many approaches in high technology heart care. I believe you will agree with the use of the word after reading this book.

Nearly half of all the deaths in this country are heart related (heart disease, stroke, atherosclerosis, etc.). Since you or someone you know will almost assuredly be faced with this problem it is to your advantage to become aware of the treatment options available and learn which ones to pursue and which ones to avoid. This book will give you an honest overview of what really works and what doesn't. It's a book you can't afford to be without.

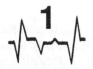

1

MEDICAL MANAGEMENT OF
CORONARY ARTERY DISEASE

An unavoidable conclusion is that the way in which our medical care system has evolved has created conditions that increase the likelihood of damage to the patient.

Rick Carlson
The End of Medicine

When heart problems strike, Americans usually find themselves under the care of a specialist. After a history and physical examination, the heart specialist can evaluate the patient further by ordering any number of sophisticated tests.

The EKG was developed in 1919. Then came tests for enzymes which pour into the blood when heart muscle cells die during a heart attack. Other tests the cardiologist can choose from are the treadmill stress test, echocardiogram, isotope scan, angiogram, PET scan, and the ultra-fast CT scan. When testing is completed a basic decision must be made between recommending a surgical procedure (bypass surgery or balloon angioplasty) or medical management.

HEART DEATH RATES ARE DOWN

Most Americans are not aware that death rates from coronary artery disease have fallen substantially in recent years. Yearly death rates for people known to have obstructions in all three of their main coronary arteries fell continually from about 11 to 2 percent between 1960 and 1985.

Most people would automatically connect the improvement in death rates with bypass surgery and balloon procedures, but there is no evidence for this conclusion. Experts give the credit to two factors: improvements individuals have made in their diets and lifestyles, and the medical management of heart attack victims in coronary care units of hospitals. The death rate had almost bottomed out before coronary bypass surgery and balloon procedures appeared on the scene.

CORONARY CARE UNITS

Cardiologists have good reason to be proud of the development of the coronary care unit, or CCU. However, as you will see, the CCU is one of the few bright spots in treatment of coronary artery disease.

The coronary care unit is a separate department in a hospital where heart patients receive specialized care from highly trained personnel. When patients enter a coronary care unit (CCU) they are immediately attached to EKG machines that run 24 hours a day. Monitors are equipped with automatic alarms, and tracings are displayed at the nursing station. When a dangerous rhythm change occurs bells go off and lights flash. Every effort is made to convert the heart beat rhythm back to one that will support an adequate pumping action.

PACEMAKERS

If patients have rhythm problems that cause the heart to beat too fast or too slow, pacemakers can be installed. The pacemaker is a battery powered device that is surgically sewn under the skin of the upper chest. A wire from the pacemaker is threaded down a vein into the heart. Pacemakers monitor the heart's rhythm. Different types of pacemakers can stimulate the heart to speed up or slow down as needed. They frequently can be life saving.

I remember a poor old fellow who attended the free clinic of my medical school when I was a student. Joe was a burned out alcoholic and street bum, the forerunner of homeless people of today. Periodically old Joe's heart would skip about ten beats in a row. When this happened blood flow to this brain stopped and he would fall flat on his face.

When he showed up at the clinic his face was usually swollen, bleeding, and discolored. It was an easy task to diagnose his problem with an electrocardiogram, but there was noting that could be done for him in 1959. We treated his bruises and sent him back to his heating grate. If pacemakers had existed, Joe could have at least stayed on his feet while sober.

As wonderful as the invention has been, not all news about pacemakers has been good. A few years ago a kickback scheme was exposed. If a surgeon installed a certain number of one company's pacemakers, a free trip for two to a tropical island was awarded as a prize. The result was that many people received pacemakers who didn't need them. One study of pacemaker implantations in Philadelphia found that 20 percent were unnecessary, another 36 percent highly questionable.

CLOT DISSOLVERS

A second emergency treatment for acute heart attacks that is proving to save lives is the use of clot dissolving drugs. Drugs such as streptokinase, Eminase, and TPA, can be injected in the vein to dissolve clots that are plugging up a heart artery and causing a heart attack.

Recent clot dissolving studies refer to a *golden hour*, the first hour after a heart attack begins. If a patient arrives at a hospital during the first hour of a heart attack, and one of these drugs is given, the risk of dying in the hospital can be reduced by over 50 percent. If given later, the drugs are less effective. Therefore, as in the case of treating abnormal rhythm problems, chances of survival are improved if patients are transported to a hospital as soon as a heart attack is suspected.

CLOT DISSOLVERS AND CRAZINESS

A side issue about these clot dissolvers demonstrates some of the ways in which vested financial interests manipulate the way medicine is practiced. Three drug companies have clot dissolvers on the market. In each case the medication is used only once, shortly after a heart attack. All work about equally well.

Tissue Plasminogen Activator, or TPA form Burroughs-Wellcome, costs about $3,500 for a single dose. A second clot dissolver, Eminase from Smith Kline Beecham, costs $1,700 per dose. A third, streptokinase, from Astra, costs about $250. According to the logic of modern medicine and excellent marketing the most expensive clot dissolver has more than 70 percent of the market share. Hospital pharmacies stock all three drugs. The choice is left to individual physicians who are never challenged about why they prescribe one drug in place of another.[1]

Physicians frequently prescribe certain drugs, or brand name drugs in place of cheaper generics, as a result of the actions of drug company salespeople. A gift of a pen and pencil set many swing the prescribing decision in a favorable direction. The decision may be maneuvered by the gift of a free weekend trip for two to a beach resort in Florida during January. Possibly the doctor's retirement plan owns stock in one of the companies. When I was a resident physician one company yearly treated all doctors in training in our department (including our dates or wives) to a carte blanch evening at Trader Vic's followed by a major league ball game. We prescribed a lot of drugs for urinary infections, that company's major products.

ANTI-ARRHYTHMIA DRUGS

Special drugs can also be used to control arrhythmia. However, problems have arisen with most anti-arrhythmia drugs in the past. Two drugs, Enkaid and Tambocor, were taken off the market in 1989 because they were found to increase the risk of heart attacks and death. Another anti-arrhythmia drug, milrinone, was under investigation in 1991 when the trial was abruptly discontinued due to a high number of deaths. A patient of mine recently had an experience with another new anti-arrhythmia medication.

Alec K. was having near fatal episodes of ventricular tachycardia. His heart was beating so rapidly (280 beats per minute) it was doing little more than quivering. This is a life threatening condition because no blood is being pumped.

Surgeons inserted a $30,000 defibrillating pacemaker into his chest. In a short period of time after surgery, the defibrillator had shocked him three times to correct abnormalities. At that point Alec's cardiologist recommended he begin taking a new drug for his rhythm problems, Cordarone (amioderone).

Alec asked his doctor for information he could read about the drug. Instead of receiving a copy of the drug's product insert (approved by the Food and Drug Administration). Alec was given a two page description of Cordarone that had been written and typed by the hospital's pharmacy. Pulmonary toxicity (lung damage) was the worst side effect listed, occurring in 2 to 4 percent of users. The problem was minimized and it was implied that side effects would clear up if the medicine was discontinued. Risk of dying from this lung complication was not mentioned.

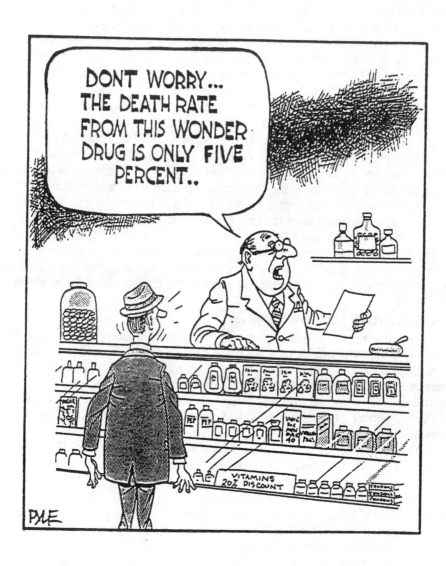

Alec asked me to get some information about the drug. A pharmacist supplied us with the FDA approved product insert. The insert contained a large black box around a warning that was printed in bold type. This *always* means bad news.

Pulmonary toxicity (lung damage) was reported to have occurred in 10 to 17 percent of people taking Cordarone in experimental studies. Among people who suffered this complication the death rate was 10 percent. Apparently, in studies required for its approval by the Food and Drug Administration, between 1 and 1.7 percent of patients who took Cordarone died of lung complications. This was quite a different picture from the hospital's deceptive version.

Other side effects listed included liver damage and a worsening of the arrhythmia. Frequently the rhythm problem is even more difficult to control for some time *after* Cordarone has been discontinued. It is a sad day when a hospital feels it must resort to deceiving patients about serious side effects of drugs it supplies. Many people wonder how Cordarone was ever approved by the FDA.

Other drugs intended for use in the treatment of coronary artery disease are not so toxic. Most are used either to treat or try to prevent angina pains. Calcium channel blockers have been quite effective in relieving the pain of angina. They work by keeping excess amounts of calcium from building up in cells, thus helping to prevent spasms that can reduce or completely shut off blood flow in coronary arteries. Nitroglycerin has been used for decades to dilate coronary arteries. Also used frequently are various beta blockers, but benefits reported in preventing heart attacks are small.

ANGIOGRAMS

Doctors began to do heart catheterizations over three decades ago. In the usual procedure a long thin catheter is inserted into the femoral artery (in the groin) and threaded up the aorta to the heart. Measurements of blood samples for gases (oxygen and carbon dioxide) and pressures in different parts of the heart are taken. These data have been indispensable in diagnosing birth defects of the heart as well as problems with heart valves.

In 1963 the first angiograms were performed. During an angiogram a catheter is passed up the aorta to a point just above the heart. A material is then injected (loosely referred to as a dye) which will flow through the arteries of the heart and show up on an X ray.

In the early days of angiograms radiologists performed the tests and interpreted the results. Cardiologists soon began to do the test on their own patients. So it was that a new breed of catheter passing cardiologist was born and launched on the road to riches. Cash registers began to clang in cardiologists' offices as decimal points in fee schedules were moved several places to the right. When the balloon angioplasty (stretching of an obstruction with a balloon) arrived on the scene, financial opportunities for cardiologists multiplied exponentially.

The angiogram was treated with awe as if it was a miraculous technique. For the first time doctors could see what the inside of the main arteries of the heart looked like as blood was rushing through them. The angiogram also created a recording on paper that doctors could hold in their hands. Seeing the results of a test on a piece of paper has become highly important to doctors. It makes a test seem more scientific, meaningful, and reassuring then it really may be.

The angiogram began to be used as a reliable indicator of the extent of obstructions in the plumbing of the heart. Cardiologists loved the test and began to refer to pictures of the arteries seen on an angiogram as a *road map*. There is just one tiny problem with the angiogram: it is a very inaccurate test.

HOW ACCURATE IS THE ANGIOGRAM?

The angiogram became well accepted and quickly spread throughout the land. Physicians were shocked when the first studies related to accuracy were published in 1974, about ten years after the first angiograms had been done. Angiograms that had been used to plan bypass surgery were compared with the actual arteries of patients who died shortly after what is commonly called *life saving* bypass surgery. *Serious* discrepancies were found.[2]

Accuracy was studied a second way at Massachusetts General Hospital in 1976 (in association with the Harvard Medical School Office of Information Technology).[3] Four experienced readers of angiograms were asked to participate in the study. Some of these physicians had been interpreting the test for nine years, and each had read a minimum of 1,500 antiograms. In addition, these doctors taught the method to other physicians in training at one of the most respected teaching hospitals in the country.

Only angiograms of the highest photographic quality were used in the study. Each expert was asked to examine a specific area of one coronary artery and report the degree of obstruction he saw as a percentage. Readings between the four experts were then compared.

Wide differences of opinion were found. In the worst cases one expert read an area of an artery as being totally blocked (100 percent), while another saw no obstruction at all (0 percent). You can't get further apart. In actual daily practice each film would be read by only one physician and a treatment regime would be based on that reading. The accuracy of angiograms is of great importance because experts recommend that only arteries more than 50 percent obstructed should be treated surgically and those less than 50 percent left alone. But which ones are they?

A third study was presented at a meeting of the American Heart Association in 1979, but never published. Thirty abnormal angiograms were circulated between three well respected medical centers for consensus evaluations. On the first time around there was significant disagreement between the readers in 39 percent of the films.

A few months later the same films were recycled through the same centers and read by the same experts. Individual radiologists were found to disagree substantially with their own previous reading 32 percent of the time. [4]

In 1984 a fourth study was published that approached the problem yet another way. Preoperative angiographic readings were compared to doppler (ultrasound) flow velocity readings taken directly on coronary arteries with the chest open during bypass surgery. The doppler readings were accepted as reliable, representing the *gold standard*.

So many discrepancies in interpretations were found the authors concluded, "The physiologic (blood flow) effects of the majority of coronary obstructions can not be determined accurately by conventional angiographic approaches. *The results of these studies should be profoundly disturbing to all physicians who have relied on the coronary arteriogram to provide accurate information regarding the physiologic consequences of individual coronary stenosis (obstruction)"* [italics mine].[5] Translated into plain English this means that the ordinary angiogram is so inaccurate it should not be used to plan bypass surgery or balloon procedures. The article even referred to the practice in the past tense as if this revelation would stop physicians from doing just that.

These studies of accuracy of the ordinary angiogram stand unopposed. After an extensive research of the medical literature I could find no articles that have reported the antiogram to be an accurate test. If such articles exist I am certain they would have been publicized to counter the negative reports referred to above.

MUM'S THE WORD

Three of these studies were published in leading medical journals. No efforts were made to attract media attention to the embarrassing results. If the media had picked up the story they could have accurately reported, "The diagnostic test used to scare the pants off heart disease patients and coerce them into billions of dollars of unnecessary surgical procedures is a scam." The information was ignored by physicians and never picked up by the press.

After these reports were published, the volume of angiograms, coronary bypass surgeries and balloon angioplasties continued to increase dramatically. In fact, during the time these reports were being made public, bypass surgeons and balloon passing cardiologists were double-shifting their steam roller into warp drive. Nothing was going to stand in their way. Now, a good 20 years later, medical schools continue to teach how to perform and read the ordinary angiogram, never mentioning its lack of accuracy.

I have shown these articles to heart patients who have had angiograms who have then questioned their own doctors as to this problem of accuracy. Some doctors replied that they were aware of the studies, but they considered the question to be moot. At their local hospital (in Missoula or Paducah), radiologists know how to read angiograms accurately (which means better than at Harvard). Arrogance is alive and well in medicine.

Most American doctors have probably never heard of these studies. Negative comments about medicine are not welcomed by doctors, and those that originate from within medicine usually are stored quietly away in medical libraries. Doctors continue to use the inaccurate angiogram as a guide in recommending surgical procedures to patients. The tactics used in these sales pitches raise questions of ethics and fraud.

WOULD YOU BUY A USED ANGIOGRAM FROM DR. JECKYL AND MR. HYDE?

The angiogram is used as a major sales device in the clinical setting. The sales pitch is similar to what goes on in used car lots, and the salespeople are just about as slick. The scene usually develops slowly. It builds up like a crescendo in music but in the finale, instead of hearing the crash of cymbals, you hear a breast bone being cracked open. In many ways it resembles a Broadway play, but it is no comedy. (The following satirical skit is based on what patients have described to me over the years. All names used are fictitious and the characters are not intended to resemble persons ripping off the system, either living or dead.)

Cast:
Prima donnas: The bypass surgeon—Dr. Cut'em-up
The cardiologist—Dr. Sadam Who-sane?
Supporting actor: Jones, a heart attack victim.
Chorus: Nurses, technicians and family members.
THE Prop: The angiogram.

Act I: The Set Up

Something scary has happened that has landed Jones (the supporting actor in more ways than one) in the hospital. Usually this means a heart attack, an episode of angina, or bad intestinal gas. A condition of high anxiety puts Jones at a decided disadvantage in this game.

After isolating the problem to the heart, Dr. Who-sane? follows his programming, automatically recommending an angiogram. He points out how important it is for doctors to see the *road map* of the plumbing of the heart. Only then can experts decide how to correct the plumbing problem and save Jones' life. Jones is wheeled off to the X-ray department as the *Death March* plays quietly in the background on the hospital's public address system.

Back in bed Joe is terrified, anxiously waiting to find out if he is ever going to get better, or even survive. He is pale, sweating, and has widely dilated pupils. He grabs the side rails of his bed and twists them into odd shapes.

Nurse Gotcha gives Jones a shot of morphine in his bare butt. This serves multiple purposes. First it lets Jones know who is in charge. The morphine also clouds his mind which makes it easier to get the surgical consent form signed.

Act II: The Sting

The co-stars of this performance (cardiologist Doctor Who-sane? and heart surgeon Dr. Cut'em-up) receive their cues and enter the hospital room wearing surgical uniforms and white hats. Dr. Who-sane? is wearing new apparel around his neck and a light reflection off of it momentarily blinds Jones.

Jones asks, "What is that around your neck, Dr. Who-sane?"

Dr. Who-sane? replies, "This gold plated heart catheter signifies I have been initiated into the million dollar club of *invasive cardiologists*. I am very proud of it."

Jones comments, "Congratulations Dr. Who-sane?"

"Thank you."

The doctors show Jones a drawing of his heart on which obstructions and percentages have been sketched in with a pencil. Members of the family are sobbing quietly in the background, expecting the worst.

Cut'em-up opens the pitch by saying, "Doctor Who-sane? and I have decided what we are going to do to you. It was a close call so we flipped a coin. I won, so you are going to have a bypass." He points to an obstruction and says, "Let's look at your *road map* here. This one's 90 percent blocked, a real *widow maker*. We had better fix this spot right away, and maybe this spot...and...mmmm...maybe this area over here. You did say you are insured with Blue Cross?"

Jones is having a hard time thinking straight because of the morphine. He asks, "Dr. Cut'em-up, "What will happen to me if I don't have a bypass?"

Cut'em-up replies, "It is very simple. You will die. If we don't get into your chest tonight and fix your plumbing problem, your heart attack will spread and you won't be alive by morning. I would also miss payments on my wife's Lamborghini and our yacht."

Jones asks, "What sort of death rate do you have with these bypasses?"

Cut'em-up avoids eye contact and lies, "Around here we say our death rate is one percent."

Jones asks, "Are there any alternatives to surgery? I've been reading about some diet and lifestyle programs. If I followed one of those plans could I avoid the surgery?"

Cut'em-up lays down his doughnut and flicks his cigarette across the room into an ash tray. "I have decided those programs are so involved and time consuming none of my patients would ever follow them. The recipes are awful. Do you want to nibble rabbit food for the rest of your life? Your only real option is to have me do the surgery, and the sooner the better. Trust me."

Jones seems to remember the last time somebody told him to trust him and he did, he lost a lot of money, but he is too drugged to think clearly. Slurring his speech he says, "O.K. sounds just peachy to me." He yanks the clip board from Cut'em-up's hand and scrawls his name on the dotted line.

"Oh, I have one last question. What are you going to do to me during the surgery?"

Cut'em-up replies slipping back into doctor-ease because the formalities of the sale are over. "First we cut out some veins form your legs and split your breast bone open with a power saw. Don't worry about that part because the saw has a guard on its tip that keeps us form cutting into you too deeply. Also, you will be happy to hear that we now wear motorcycle helmets and visors to protect us from getting AIDS from you. We crank your ribs open with a ratchet. We hook one end of each vein to your aorta and sew the other end to a coronary artery with end-to-side anastomoses. While this is going on you will be on the heart lung machine and monitored for everything from cardiac output to arterial rhubarb concentration. When you wake up you will have a tube in your throat as big as a fire hose. In five days I will send you home."

Jones says, "I, I, I've heard that before."

Cut'em-up replies arrogantly, "You haven't heard it from me before!"

A clerk from the admitting department enters the room and announces that Jones' medical insurance is in good shape. The billing department has turned on the green light. Led by the prima donnas, everybody breaks into a happy chorus of harmony, praising the angiogram and bypass, and they all live happily ever after (at least the doctors do). Little does Jones know he has just bought a lemon—The End.

A new lingo has been created for these sales pitches. Even female patients are told they have widow makers. The term is used generically. I have never heard of a female patient being told she has a *widower* maker. Other people have been told they have a serious blockage, or that their life is hanging by a thread.

Other patients have been frightened out of their hospital gowns when doctors have told them they are living with a time bomb, have a tight obstruction, critical obstruction, high grade lesion, or jeopardized myocardium. Usually a coronary artery bypass surgery or angioplasty is recommended as being absolutely necessary to get them through the next few days, alive.

These are scenes of high drama and the prima donnas are skilled at manipulating the outcome. If you ever find yourself playing the role of Jones in a skit like this you should ask to see the doctors' membership cards in the actor's union. Then again, that would be a waste of time. No respectable heart surgeon would degrade himself by showing his membership card to a lowly patient.

ESCAPE FROM THE HOSPITAL

Geogre G. described how these intimidating tactics were used on him. He was shown drawings of his obstructions and told he had a real widow maker in one spot. The bypass surgeon told him, "If we don't improve the blood flow to your heart immediately, you will not be alive by tomorrow morning. If you don't agree to the surgery I will not be responsible for what happens to you."

George was adamant in refusing surgery. During the next four hours he had to repeat his refusal about twenty times as various physicians, nurses, and counselors came to his bedside to convince him to have the operation. As he described it, he finally escaped from the hospital by signing the *against medical advice* form.

George went on a natural food diet, took some vitamins and minerals, and started chelation treatments. He is alive and free of symptoms thirteen years later.

There are additional problems with angiograms that create problems of accuracy. Coronary arteries sometimes go into spasm and contract when a catheter or dye material is injected into them. This will affect the film and lead to an overestimation of obstruction. Another problem is that X-ray pictures are taken with just one camera. If an artery opening is flat, the amount of obstruction seen on the X ray will vary according to the angle from which the picture is taken.

Another problem is that collateral circulation will not show on an angiogram unless the vessels are quite large. Collaterals are the body's way of building detour routes around arteries as obstructions slowly begin to form. If collaterals are substantial, circulation adequate enough to keep tissues alive can be maintained, even if the main artery is 100 percent obstructed. These examples may explain some variability in measurements, but they don't answer why experts at Harvard and other centers interpreted identical angiograms so differently.

An additional problem is that the angiogram carries a major risk all of its own. For every 1,000 angiograms performed, about one person dies from a complication directly related to the procedure. Frequently a potentially fatal heart rhythm is triggered by nothing more than the presence of the dye in the artery.

QUANTITATIVE ANGIOGRAMS

By the 1970s many researchers were writing that a more accurate method of measuring blockages in the coronary arteries was needed. Researchers had been avoiding using the angiogram as a means of following the long term course of coronary artery disease because of the accuracy problem.

In 1977, B. Greg Brown described a new angiographic technique he called *quantitative angiography.* Views of coronary arteries are taken from two angles simultaneously with two cameras to achieve a three dimensional effect. Data are interpreted by a computer, not the human eye ball. The method measures diameters of arteries accurately to within 150 microns, producing a margin of error of only 1 percent.[6] This distinguishes it from the conventional or *ordinary angiogram*, the term I like to use for the commonly available, inaccurate procedure.

By the mid 1980s a few university medical centers were using the technique, but generally only for research. The average doctor and the general public have almost no access to the method. Its very existence has almost been veiled like an industrial trade secret. You can rest assured when an angiogram is being advised to you, you will not be told of the differences between these two methods, nor about the inaccuracy of the test commonly offered.

Other researchers have used variations of this three dimensional technique. Sometimes they have failed to report that the method they are using is different than the ordinary angiogram. This represents a form of deception which is probably intended to keep ordinary rank and file physicians from learning about the differences in angiograms and becoming upset.

One such article was published in the *Journal of the American Medical Association* titled, "Changes in Sequential Coronary Angiograms and Subsequent Coronary Events." Translated into English the title means that several coronary angiograms were taken in the same patients over a period of time to evaluate the effectiveness of a treatment procedure. In this case the treatment being evaluated was a surgical procedure that reduced bowel length with the intent of reducing blood cholesterol levels (researchers do take this cholesterol business far more seriously than they should as you will see in Chapter 5).

The method of engiography used was not described either in the title or the text. The article contained a statement that the "evaluation protocol (for the angiogram) was virtually identical to that used by the Cholesterol Lowering Atherosclerotic Study."[7] It would have taken fewer words to say that a form of quantitative angiography had been used.

Instead, the reader was referred to reference article number 10 that was published in a rather obscure research journal most hospital libraries don't stock.

When I asked a hospital medical librarian to obtain that article for me I was charged $5 for the service and had to wait two weeks for delivery. Only then did I confirm my suspicion that a form of quantitative angiography had been used. This certainly was not made clear in the original article.[8]

I saw a patient who brought in reports of two different angiograms. The first angiogram, of ordinary pedigree, was performed in a neighborhood hospital. Vince had suffered a heart attack which had damaged a significant amount of muscle tissue. The angiogram revealed no obstructions in the artery that led to the part of his heart that other tests had shown to be damaged. This bothered his doctors.

A few months later Vince underwent a quantitative angiogram in a university medical center. That angiogram showed a major obstruction where the doctors suspected one should be from the beginning. The physicians told him only that the first angiogram had *missed* the obstruction. The blockage had obviously been there for a long time.

It is obvious that there was no reason to do the second angiogram. A decision had already been made that Vince was not a candidate for bypass surgery or a balloon procedure because of the extent of damage to his heart muscle (a low ejection fraction of 30%). The second angiogram appears to have been done solely to satisfy the curiosity of the university specialists. Vince was exposed to a risky procedure for nothing.

This points out a problem that frequently arises in modern medicine. When a doctor recommends a test that carries with it a significant risk, it is wise to ask how the test might provide information that is useful to the management of you own condition. For example, if you are adamantly opposed to having a bypass surgery or balloon procedure, then there is no reason in the world to submit to an angiogram.

I have never been one to believe in conspiracy stories concerning medical therapies and their suppression. However, I would not be surprised if there is a covert game plan functioning here. The ordinary angiogram will be replaced with the quantitative method quietly and slowly with as few people knowing about the change as possible. This does appear to be happening as a commercially available instrument is now on the market.

The quantitative angiogram represents a giant step forward. It gives researchers a way to measure the effects of treatment efforts on obstructed areas of arteries. However, I am shocked because of what has not happened. This new technique should have been announced publicly as a major improvement and breakthrough. Such a revelation would have publicly exposed the ordinary angiogram for what it is. But, if that had happened, the multibillion dollar a year bypass and balloon industries would have been torpedoed in their underbellies. Therefore, vested interests have had good reasons to suppress information about the quantitative angiogram.

SUMMARY

Medical management of coronary artery disease has its bright spots and blemishes. Specialized coronary care units have saved many lives by successfully treating arrhythmias and other crisis situations that frequently arise in the first few days following a heart attack. Clot dissolving drugs also show promise in this regard. By contrast, the use of anti-arrhythmia drugs continues to be associated with high rates of serious and frequently fatal complications.

The only studies made public to date to measure accuracy of the ordinary angiogram have demonstrated serious problems with the method. An accurate form of angiography exists, but it is usually used only for research purposes. Few doctors or patients have access to these machines because only a handful exist. Not informing patients about the inaccuracy of the ordinary angiogram deserves to be called a fraud on the public.

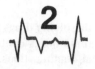

2

OF CABBAGES AND THEIR KINGS

The unkindest cut of all is when a doctor performs unnecessary surgery (on you).

Anonymous

George Jones collapsed in his office with crushing chest pain and was rushed to the hospital. The high tech tools of modern medicine were mobilized into action. George's internist quickly diagnosed a heart attack and ordered an angiogram. The angiogram showed serious obstructions in the arteries of his heart and bypass surgery was recommended.

A heart surgeon was called in. The surgeon described how pieces of veins from George's legs would be used to detour blood around areas of obstruction in the main arteries of his heart, thus improving blood flow to his ailing heart muscle.

Because heart disease ran in his family, George had read extensively on the subject. He asked the surgeon what would happen in two to five years when the bypass veins usually close off. The chest surgeon replied casually, "Well, when you have more trouble we can take you back to surgery and do another bypass."

This story exemplifies the current philosophical approach modern medicine applies to coronary artery disease. The heart attack is viewed primarily as a plumbing problem. The quick fix is to call in a bunch of would be plumbers to install some new pipes as detours.

The coronary bypass operation stands as a monument to an almost total lack of understanding of causes, prevention, and effective management of this disease. The only large scale studies ever conducted to try to prove that bypass surgery extends life showed it doesn't. Heart patients lived just as long without the surgery. But this is not what most people (and doctors) believe.

A LITTLE HISTORY

In the early part of this century medical management of coronary artery disease was simple. Angina pains were treated with nitroglycerin tablets which were dissolved under the tongue. When a heart attack struck, treatment consisted of prolonged bed rest and morphine for pain. Basically, patients were on their own. They either made it or they didn't.

Thirty-five years ago little was known about what to expect after a heart attack. My father died of a heart attack in 1958 during my freshman year in medical school. The subject became personal and I have followed changes in the field ever since. When our pathology professor assigned a term paper, a classmate and I decided to research survival after a heart attack. This classmate now is a coronary bypass surgeon.

Harry and I went to the school library to see what we could find. The first revelation was that papers on survival after heart attacks didn't exist in American medical journals. We were lucky to find a mere five reports from Scandinavian countries. As students this was serendipity. Researching the subject was so easy we had a little more time to drink beer.

A consistent pattern emerged. About 40 percent of people died with their first heart attack, either before or after arriving at the hospital. Survivors lived an average of five more years, had another heart attack, and again 40 percent of them died. Survivors lived an average of three more years, had another heart attack, and again 40 percent died. Survivors lived another two years, had another heart attack, an again 40 percent died. This left few survivors by ten years.

In the 1960s survival rates began to improve. The death rate for patients with disease in all three of their main coronary arteries had been running 11.4 percent per year. By the mid 1970s the death rate had fallen to 4.8 percent. By the late 1970s it was 3.5 percent. By the early 1980s it had fallen to 2.1 percent per year, a level so low it is impossible to improve upon with invasive surgical procedures.

SURGEONS RUSH IN WHERE ANGLES...

In the 1950s surgeons were more than happy to help in the search for treatments for coronary artery disease. An old joke goes that surgeons know nothing but do everything. In they jumped.

The fad surgical procedure for angina at the time involved tying off the internal mammary arteries. The internal mammary arteries run vertically down our chests just inside the ribs on each side of the breast bone (sternum). This procedure was based on the assumption that if some arteries were tied off near the heart, more blood might find its way through plugged coronary arteries. There was no way to measure these blood flows at the time, so the hypothesis could not be evaluated objectively. As humans can get along without these particular arteries, they were volunteered.

The surgical procedure was simple. Surgeons made small incisions between ribs on each side of the breast bone and tied off the arteries. After the procedure it was commonplace for patients to find themselves free of pain, then boast about how much their surgeons had done for them. Surgeons are not immune to that kind of stroking and it led to more procedures.

In several studies, about 36 percent of patients reported relief of angina symptoms following this operation. When additional studies confirmed these findings, the lay press popularized the procedure in authoritative sources of medical information such as *Reader's Digest*. Because doctors had nothing else to offer at the time, the procedure had no competition and spread rapidly like the flu.

One day a funny thing happened on the way back from the operating room. A surgical team that was dead tired from being up all night was scheduled to perform one of these operations in the morning. The patient was taken to surgery, sedated, and the incisions were made. Everyone in the operating room must have been asleep or day dreaming because the surgeons forgot to tie off the arteries and nobody noticed.

By the time the omission was discovered it was too late. The patient was regaining his senses in the recovery room. It's awkward for a surgeon to tell a patient nobody remembered to do his operation and everyone should be nice about this and quietly return to the operating room for another try.

Surprisingly, the patient reported complete relief of his chest pains. This stroke of luck saved the surgeons the agony of defeat, telling the patient they had forgotten to do his surgery. This presumes their intent was to be honest with the patient, which is probably expecting too much.

The story exists as a rumor and was never published, which is not surprising. Physicians normally don't write papers about their errors in judgment and publish them in the underground medical journal titled *Ooops*. I have never seen articles with titles such as, "How I cut the Leg Off of the Wrong Patient (But it Was the Nurse's Fault)" or "How I Took Out the Patient's Only Kidney But is was an Honest Mistake." These reports appear in newspaper articles related to malpractice suits.

This story about forgetting to do the surgery spread verbally and raised doubts about the usefulness of tying off internal mammary arteries. A study was planned to evaluate the procedure.

Seventeen patients were scheduled to have the surgery. Patients were randomized to receive either the real operation or merely skin incisions. The investigators were true to the scientific method. The victims were not informed they were going to participate in the first and only controlled study of a surgical procedure in the history of medicine.

A similar study would be impossible to perform today because of medical ethics committees that oversee human experimentation. That was not a problem in 1959. No one was looking over the doctors' shoulders.

When results were published a shock wave shot through the surgical community. The rate of relief of angina was the same in patients who had their arteries tied off as those who received only skin incisions. This was correctly interpreted as showing that the benefits reported from the surgery were nothing more than a placebo response. The procedure died almost overnight.[1]

The next surgical procedure intended to relieve the pain of angina originated from another theory of how to increase circulation to the heart muscle. The heart is covered with a thin slippery surface called the pericardium. This well lubricated surface allows the heart to move freely as it contracts and expands. Surgeons speculated that if they roughed up this slippery surface, new blood vessels might grow across to the area of the heart that was not getting enough blood. Once again glowing results were claimed. Many patients said their angina went away completely.

I saw a variation of the procedure when I was in my residency training. The sack surrounding the heart was opened and talcum powder was puffed in. Surgeons hoped an abrasive action would stimulate blood vessel growth on the outside of the heart. This procedure never became widespread and eventually disappeared. A lot of people had their chests opened for nothing.

An even more bizarre procedure was the Vineberg operation which experienced a brief period of popularity in the early 1960s. Surgeons cut off one end of the internal mammary artery and stuffed the free end into a puncture hole made in the heart muscle with a tool resembling an ice pick (perhaps it really was an ice pick). Proponents hoped this large artery would mysteriously develop connections with tiny arteries in the heart. The amazing thing is that such a connection apparently did grow in the heart of one animal that received the operation.

As usual, surgeons claimed great success. However, these pronouncements never had a chance to be verified because a new procedure arrived on the scene that looked better. This was coronary artery bypass surgery, officially known as the Coronary Artery Bypass Graft (or Grafting). The procedure is abbreviated as CABG, and referred to routinely and affectionately in medical slang as *cabbage*, the term we will henceforth use. However, two other procedures had to be developed before cabbage surgeries were possible: the coronary angiogram and the heart lung machine.

THE ANGIOGRAM

The angiogram (literally vessel view) allowed physicians to see blood flowing through the arteries of the heart. Doctors referred to X-ray pictures of these arteries as showing the *road map* of blood flow through the heart. Areas of obstructions could be identified in the arteries for the first time. Armed with this information surgeons decided where to place their detour pipes. By the time inaccuracies of the angiogram were discovered the procedure was in wide spread use. When the bad news arrived it was ignored and had no effect.

In the garden variety cabbage surgery, veins are harvested from somewhere else in the body, usually the legs. One end of a vein is connected to a fresh blood supply (the aorta) while the other is connected to the obstructed artery at a point past the blockage. The vein literally bypasses, or detours, around the obstructed area. No attempt is made to do anything to the diseased segment of artery which is left in place.

A single cabbage (bypass) operation may involve the placement of one or more grafts (detours). More recently, surgeons are swinging down the internal mammary artery as a detour around obstructions in coronary arteries. This does seem to be a more logical step, asking an artery to do the work of an artery.

I am amazed to discover how little many cabbage patients know about what has been done inside their chests. Many believe that diseased arteries have been reamed out, removed, or replaced, permanently fixing the problem. Some have said, "After all, the surgery cost enough to expect this." With total costs of an uncomplicated cabbage running anywhere from $25,000 to $75,000, they may have a point.

Deep down in their hearts bypass surgeons think like plumbers. It was natural for them to become ecstatic over the procedure. At the completion of a cabbage surgery they could take blood flow measurements with instruments and document increased blood flow downstream from the obstructions. This reinforced their expectations of what the surgery should accomplish. Most patients who were having angina also reported a relief of chest pains following the surgery.

A natural assumption is that if blood flow can be shown to be increased, then patients obviously should live longer after their plumbing repair than without it. Heart surgeons were so confident about their cabbage procedure they were willing to participate in three major controlled studies designed to see if this widely accepted conclusion was indeed correct.

THE VETERANS STUDY (1977)

The first comparison study involved 686 patients in thirteen Veterans Administration hospitals. After being randomly assigned to two groups, similar patients received either cabbage surgery or medical management.

At the end of eleven years, 58 percent of cabbage patients were alive compared to 57 percent of those treated medically. Patients who had obstructions in their left main coronary arteries had a slightly better survival rate at seven years with surgery. However, by eleven years there was no difference in survival rates between the two groups.[2]

This paper appeared in the popular and highly trusted *New England Journal of Medicine*. The day it arrived news of the disappointing results of cabbage surgery spread quickly through the medical community like the vibrations from an earthquake. Heart surgeons went into a state of shock. All over the country they were seen walking through hospital hallways with frowns on their faces. Their eyes looked dull and glazed as if they had just been hit in the side of the head with a two by four.

Everyone was whispering, "Hey, did you hear that bypass doesn't work?" Behind heart surgeons' backs some physicians had the audacity to compare this report to the terminal events that killed off the old internal mammary artery procedure. However, the report had no impact on the frequency of the operation. By this time belief patterns surrounding the surgery were too well entrenched. The procedure had become accepted with a religious fervor.

Eleven year survival curves for patients managed either surgically or medically are seen in Figure 1.

Eugene Braunwald, professor of medicine at Harvard Medical School, discussed these results in an editorial that accompanied the veterans study. Braunwald quoted a group of cardiovascular surgeons who had concluded, "This (coronary artery bypass graft) is the first operation for coronary heart disease which holds promise for improving long-term survival, and we can anticipate that it will be even more widely applied in the future for the vast numbers of people *without* angina who have advanced artherosclerotic coronary artery disease and are at risk for life-threatening myocardial infarction (heart attack) and sudden death."

Braunwald pointed out that an increasing number of patients were being operated upon, not because of the presence of intractable angina, but because of the hope, "largely without objective supporting evidence at present, that coronary bypass surgery prolongs life or diminishes the frequency of subsequent heart attack." He

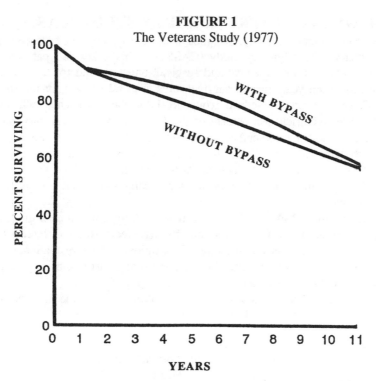

FIGURE 1
The Veterans Study (1977)

Source: *New England Journal of Medicine* 1977; 311:1333-1339.

further stated that this "rapidly growing enterprise is developing a momentum and constituency of its own, and as time passes, it will be progressively more difficult and costly to curtail it materially, if the results of carefully designed studies of its efficacy prove this step to be necessary."[3]

Top name cabbage surgeons couldn't bring themselves to believe results of the veterans study and remained convinced that cabbage surgery must extend life. Deep down in their hearts they *knew* that *their* cabbage surgery patients just had to be doing better than those managed medically. They attacked the veterans study because the operative death rate of 5.6 percent seemed too high, assuming this was the result of second rate surgery at a lowly VA hospital (care at VA hospitals is viewed as marginal by academic physicians and those in private practice).

They clamored for another study in which participating surgeons would be selected from the cream of the crop, the best in the country. In more expert hands the operative death rate should be lower. This should improve long term survival rates and make the procedure look better.

Even if such a study *could* produce results these surgeons dreamed of, it remains obscure how this might benefit an ordinary patient. The veterans study appears to have been very relevant to what could be expected to occur in the ordinary setting in which ordinary patients would receive cabbages from ordinary run-of-the-mill heart surgeons.

THE CORONARY ARTERY SURGERY STUDY (CASS)

The second comparison study, designed with the top surgeons' goals in mind, was the Coronary Artery Surgery Study (CASS). In this study 780 patients were randomized into two groups, medical and surgical, and followed for ten years.

At the end of ten years overall survival rates were 82 percent for the surgical group and 79 percent for the medical group. In the group of patients with normal function of the left ventricle (82 percent of the total group), ten year survival was 86 percent in the medical group and 82 percent in the surgical group (Figure 2). This difference was statistically significant. In patients with impaired function of the left ventricle, ten year survival was 59 percent in the medical group and 80 percent in the surgical group. This difference was not statistically significant because of the small number involved.[4]

The surgical group had less chest pain, fewer activity limitations and required less therapy with drugs at five years, but by ten years these differences had disappeared. There also was no difference in employment or recreational status between medical and surgical groups. For a second time a large study had failed to demonstrate that patients do better with cabbage surgery.[5]

What did emerge from the study was the observation that if the function of the left ventricle is normal, patients do well without surgery.

FIGURE 2
Survival in Patients with Normal Pumping
Action of the Heart

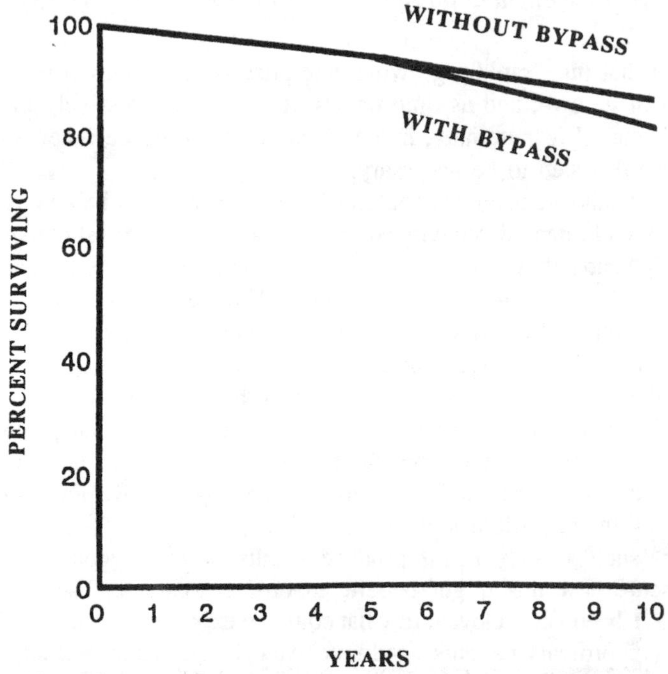

Source: Graph constructed from Alderman, et al., *Circulation* 1990; 82:1629-1646.

THE EUROPEAN STUDY (ECSSG)

The third and last large randomized study ever conducted to try to show that cabbage helps patients was the European Coronary Surgery Study Group. In patients with an abnormal EKG at rest, certain abnormalities on their treadmill tests, peripheral artery disease, or increasing age, the survival rate was better with surgery.

Researchers wrote that in the absence of these predictive variables, "the outlook is so good that early surgery is unlikely to increase the prospect of survival."[6] Once again a concept emerged that doctors could identify patients with known coronary artery disease who will do well without surgical procedures.

After summarizing these studies, professor Braunwald offered more comments about indications for cabbage surgery. He wrote, "I believe that this operation should and increasingly will be restricted to patients in whom intensive medical therapy has failed, or in whom improved survival after surgery has been unambiguously demonstrated, rather than as a panacea for coronary artery disease."[7]

Regardless of his optimism in 1983, fears Braunwald expressed in 1977 came true. An industry appeared on the scene with a remarkable growth curve. In 1975 there were 60,000 cabbage surgeries performed in the United States. In 1987 there were 230,000. By 1990 the number had risen to 380,000. According to the American Heart Association 598,000 cabbage surgeries were performed in 1995, the latest statistics available as of 1999.

Another reason for saying cabbage surgery does not do much is that by the time cabbages appeared on the scene, the death rate from coronary artery disease had already fallen dramatically because of other factors. This relationship is shown in Figure 3, along with the rapidly accelerating number of balloon procedures. As you

FIGURE 3

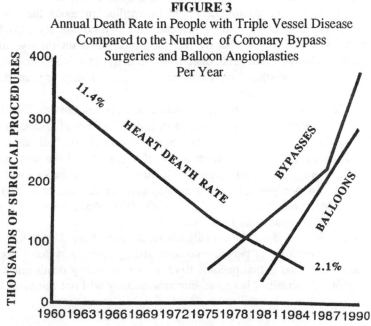

Annual Death Rate in People with Triple Vessel Disease Compared to the Number of Coronary Bypass Surgeries and Balloon Angioplasties Per Year

will see later, possibly as many as 80 to 85 percent of cabbage surgeries are not necessary, and many cabbages do more harm than good.

IT DOESN'T PAY TO CRITICIZE A MEDICAL CENTER'S BREAD AND BUTTER PROCEDURE

Dr. Henry McIntosh was an early critic of cabbage surgery. McIntosh was working in the cardiology section of Methodist Hospital at Baylor College of Medicine when the first cabbage surgery was performed in 1964. In 1978 he wrote an exhaustive 26 page summary of cabbage surgery over the previous ten years.

McIntosh wrote, "Despite a low operative mortality and rate of graft closure, available data in the literature do not indicate that myocardial infarctions (heart attacks), arrhythmias (abnormal rhythms), or congestive heart failure (failure of the heart as a pump) will be prevented, or that life will be prolonged in the vast majority of patients."[8]

Shortly after this negative paper on cabbage surgery was published, McIntosh was forced to leave his position at Baylor.

CABBAGE COMPLICATIONS

Cabbage surgery is certainly not minor surgery (minor surgery is surgery performed on someone else). The procedure carries with it a high rate of death and serious complications. If cabbage surgery is recommended, it is wise to know exactly what may lie ahead in the way of complications.

Death

Certainly the most obvious risk of cabbage surgery is death. In my area of the country prospective patients are routinely told by cardiac surgeons that, in their hands, the operative death rate is only 1 percent. This is a commonly used figure around the country, regardless of what the real facts are. When such a low number is used it is almost always a deliberate distortion. Actually, most cabbage surgeons probably don't even know what their death rates are and, if they are smart, they won't make any effort to find out.

Other sources reveal a different picture than this 1 percent answer. Five major teaching hospitals in Philadelphia participated in a death rate study. Over a thirty month period 4,613 coronary bypass surgeries were performed. Individual heart surgeons had death rates that ranged from a low of 1 percent all the way up to 9 percent.[9] And these are the rates for surgeons who are regarded as experts and teach the procedure to younger physicians. By comparison, in the veterans study the overall death rate was 5.6 percent and in California 30,000 cabbages were performed in 1989 with an overall death rate of 5.7 percent.

It has been said that if a cabbage surgeon really does have a very low death rate, he is operating on a lot of people who have strong hearts and don't need the operation. The bottom line is that patients have no way to verify death rate claims of cardiac surgeons. If hospitals have this information they will not release it to the public either.

Thomas Moore reported a horror story about cabbage surgery in his book, *Heart Failure*.[10] At the University of California Medical Center in Sacramento, a major teaching institution, the operative death rate was running about 50 percent in the late 1970s. It didn't take long for local cardiologists to notice that large numbers of patients they were referring to the medical center for cabbages were quietly leaving the hospital out the back door in boxes. Referrals for cabbage surgery slowed to a trickle.

When the hospital administration investigated to find out why the number of patients admitted for cabbage surgery was falling (and income was declining), surgeons offered their typical response. They said much sicker patients were being referred to their medical center than to other university medical centers. As usual this did not turn out to be the case.

Eventually the University fired all of its cabbage surgeons. The conflicts ended up in legal charges, counter charges, and slander suits. A whole group of new cabbage surgeons was hired. Under new management the operative death rate soon fell to levels seen in similar institutions, the number of cases admitted went up, and everyone was happy again.

Where did the cabbage surgeons with the high death rates go? You can be certain they didn't consider themselves to be examples of the *Peter Principle* and retire for the sake of humanity. Prima donnas with hyperinflated egos would never do that. They moved on to practice their trade in other fertile pastures, perhaps one is operating in your community.

This horror story demonstrates one of the ongoing problems in medicine. Modern medicine has never developed a means of monitoring itself adequately enough to protect the public. In the cabbage surgery area this would not be a difficult task.

Insurance companies already know which surgeons have high complication rates and which ones don't. Insurance companies keep longitudinal records on their clients. A simple computer cross check could identify surgeons whose patients die too frequently, or require extended hospital stays because of complications. In many states these statistics are monitored as well. It would be in everyone's best interests if this information became public. Possibly it would take some sort of freedom of information action to release information gathered by states. Of course, heart surgeons would automatically rise up and lobby against such as action.

More Rapid Closure of Arteries and Grafts

Another problem with cabbages became apparent quite early. It was found that the rate of formation of additional obstruction in *native* arteries increased rapidly in some patients (a native artery is an artery you are born with). This problem is related to flow dynamics through arteries and the inaccuracy of angiogram readings.

Blood flow will not be reduced in an artery until there is at least a 75 percent obstruction in the channel through which it is passing. Up to that point the same amount of blood can pass through an obstruction simply by speeding up. Because of the mathematics of calculating the surface area of a circle (Pi multiplied by the radius squared) it becomes critical to know if an artery is obstructed more or less than 50 percent. A 50 percent reduction in diameter will produce a 75 percent reduction in the opening in an artery. At that point blood flow will begin to be reduced.

With a routine angiogram, arteries with less than a 50 percent obstruction are frequently interpreted as being more obstructed, then surgically bypassed. When that happens much more blood than is needed flows to the tissues past the obstruction. The body compensates for this unwanted increase in flow by closing down the native artery at an accelerated rate, said to be 1,000 percent faster than it was becoming obstructed before the surgery.

It also is reported that obstructions form in grafted veins faster than in native arteries. Post operative angiograms sometimes have shown cabbage grafts to be totally obstructed within two weeks after surgery.

Complications from the Heart-Lung Machine

Use of the heart-lung machine is associated with its own complications. During cabbage surgery the heart must be stopped at the beginning of the surgery, then restarted after all of the grafts are in place. There doesn't seem to be any way to prevent blood flow to the brain from being reduced substantially during this process, even in the best of hands.

In one study from Sweden, 12 percent of cabbage patients had obvious brain damage from the surgery, such as strokes. However, *all* of the other patients showed marked disturbances on intellectual tests given two months after surgery as compared to tests before surgery.[11]

This loss of intellectual ability is also seen in patients who have been placed on the heart-lung machine for operations other than cabbage surgery. Therefore, it appears the problem is caused by a reduced flow of oxygen to the brain that is related to the use of the machine, not to the cabbage surgery itself. Unfortunately, cabbage surgery can't be done without using a heart-lung machine.

Blood Transfusions

Another possible complication from cabbage surgery is related to blood transfusions. The heart-lung machine must be primed with several pints of blood or other fluid. When blood is used cabbage patients may be exposed to blood borne diseases, such as AIDS and hepatitis B.

Prior to 1983 surgeons used about six pints of donated blood to prime the heart-lung machine. After the AIDS epidemic accelerated in the United States, cabbage surgeons began to prime the heart-lung machine with saline solution (a salt water solution). This leaves patients markedly anemic after surgery, but the risk of blood borne diseases is reduced.

An example of this problem is the case of former professional tennis star, Arthur Ashe. In 1992 Ashe's privacy was invaded and he was forced to reveal that he had tested positive for the AIDS virus. He had become infected from *tainted* blood he received when he had cabbages in 1977 and 1983. Ashe died of AIDS related pneumonia in 1993.

Other Complications
In addition to the above, all of the usual surgical complications are possible with cabbage surgery. Fairly commonly seen are post-operative infections, failure of the breast bone to grow back together, chronic pain in the incision, abnormalities in the heart's rhythm, heart attacks, strokes, leaking at the sites where bypass graft vessels are attached, bleeding at other sites, transfusion reactions and poor wound healing.

HOW DOES CABBAGE SURGERY RELIEVE PAIN?
Most doctors agree cabbage surgery frequently relieves angina pains. A debate continues about how pain might be relieved. It is likely that several mechanisms may cause relief of pain.

Surgeons obviously favor the explanation that blood flow has been increased to the heart muscle. The best proof they have of this is doppler (ultrasound) flow velocity measurements taken immediately after the bypass grafts have been connected and the heart beat is restored.

Another possibility is that nerves that carry pain signals from the heart are cut during the surgery. When these nerves grow back in six to twelve months the pain may return, if that is the reason the pain was relieved with the cabbage.

Heart surgeons have an answer for recurrent problems. The surgery can be repeated, again and again. Some patients have been taken to surgery as many as five times for cabbage surgery. Usually, by that point, they die, or have run out of donor blood vessels and health insurance. Most are in such poor health they are told they would die on the operating table if another cabbage was attempted. It is likely many of these people didn't need cabbage surgery in the first place. It takes a strong heart to survive multiple surgical procedures.

A ZIPPER IN YOUR FUTURE?
At a specialty meeting a few years ago heart surgeons were presented with a remedy for the problem of repeat cabbages. An equipment manufacturer announced the development of a zipper that could be sewn into the middle of the breast bone at the time of the first cabbage. When additional procedures were performed all the surgeon had to do was make a skin incision and unzip.

A news magazine for physicians reported that heart surgeons welcomed the idea. I don't think the device ever appeared on the market, but the story demonstrates how cabbage surgeons feel about their favorite surgical procedure.

A SEA OF CABBAGES
An outspoken critic is Thomas A. Preston, professor of medicine at the University of Washington, Seattle. Preston claims fully one half of all cabbage surgeries performed in the United States are unnecessary. He says that survival rates are basically the same as with medical management, except for a well-defined minority of patients, and in most cases cabbage surgery is no more effective than a placebo.[12]

A study from the UCLA medical school calculated that only 56 percent of cabbage operations were justified according to the criteria used. In a survey of different hospitals the rate of justified cabbages varied from 37 to 78 percent.[13]

PST...HEY MEESTER. YOU WANT A BYPSS?

An example of the overutilization of cabbage surgery surfaced in the late 1970s in Phoenix, Arizona. Aggressive cabbage surgeons were enamored with the belief that cabbage surgery was *the* answer to plumbing problems in the heart. All men over 50 were advised to drop by their friendly community hospital and get an angiogram. In cases where significant obstructions were found, surgeons recommended and performed what they called a *preventive cabbage.*

No evidence has ever suggested this would be in the best interests of patients. Fortunately the practice failed to spread and faded away. Once again this experience illustrates how heart surgeons *believe* in their bread and butter operation.

THE *INSTANT* BYPASS OR BALLOON JOB

About 15 years ago a small number of heart surgeons pioneered what could be called the *instant* bypass. The recipe for an instant bypass is this: Take an available operating room. Mix in a cardiac surgeon with a little time on his hands and a heart patient with good medical insurance. Voila!

The thinking was that if blood flow to a jeopardized area of heart muscle could be improved soon after a heart attack begins, spread of the heart attack to healthy muscle could be prevented. Unfortunately, this concept was based on nothing more than wishful thinking.

In centers that push *instant* procedures the entire evaluation protocol is condensed. A patient may enter the emergency room with chest pain and have the chest incision made, all within two to three hours. I wouldn't be too surprised to find that different heart centers have competitions with prizes going to the team with the fastest time (with wagering of course). I once participated in an unpublicized competition to see who could do the fastest hysterectomy skin to skin (winning time was twenty-two minutes).

The National Institutes of Health sponsored a study on this instant approach called the Thrombolysis (clot dissolving) in Myocardial Infarction (heart attack) trial, which was abbreviated to TIMI II. A conclusion was, "Most American cardiologists have assumed that angioplasty or bypass surgery is necessary to prevent recurrent infarction (heart attack) and death caused by the coronary-artery stenoses (obstructions) that usually persist after successful thrombolytic (clot dissolving) therapy. The results of TIMI II indicate that this in *not* the case."[14]

Again an aggressive approach to coronary artery disease was found to bring no benefit. The NIH study was published in 1989 and has had no impact in centers that sell the instant cabbage or balloon approach. I continue to see patients who are being told they will be dead by morning if they don't have their cabbage or balloon job *right now.*

THE MATTER OF MONEY

Insurance coverage can affect the odds of having an invasive heart procedure. Privately insured patients were found to be 80 percent more likely to receive an angiogram than Medicaid (welfare) patients. Medicaid generally pays only a small fraction of usual and customary doctor fees, and many physicians refuse to accept such patients. Private patients were 40 percent more likely to receive a cabbage surgery and 28 percent more likely to have a balloon procedure.[15]

BARBERS AND SURGEONS

During one of my trips to China I was introduced to the chief of surgery of a large hospital in Beijing, part of the system of Western hospitals. The surgeon related to me how he had been trained to do cabbage surgery in New York and had done several bypasses after his return to China. He stopped doing the procedure because he observed that patients didn't do any better with the bypass than without.

The surgeon told me some details about how medicine functions in China. He was paid a salary of about $50 US per month (in 1987). Surgical patients were shaved before surgery by a local barber who worked on a free enterprise basis. The barber was paid a certain fee per patient and made more money than the bypass surgeon. This may be a form of poetic justice. Hundreds of years ago in Europe, all of the surgeons were barbers, and they weren't paid much.

FOLLOW THE MONEY

During the Watergate investigation, the mystery figure *Deep Throat* advised investigative reporters to *follow the money* if they wanted to understand what was going on. Financial factors play a major role in the utilization of cabbage surgery, so the same advice applies.

In Europe surgeons are paid on a salary basis. Therefore, doing more surgery means the doctor must work harder for the same amount of money. In Europe the incidence of cabbage surgery is 75 percent less than in America. A similar pattern is seen in the United States in Veterans Administration hospitals where doctors are paid a salary.

OH, YOU DON'T HAVE THE MONEY?

A patient of mine, Don D., told me a story that demonstrates the economics involved in this business. It also shows how doctors treat patients after they have been identified as having a specific problem.

Don was a rancher, a known heart patient with a history of cabbage surgery. One hot summer day Don got all hot and sweaty chasing a large bull that had escaped. He became dehydrated and weak. His heart rate slowed down to 40 beats per minute.

His wife drove him to town to see his cardiologist. The cardiologist ignored his new problem and approached him as if he had *coronary artery disease* tattooed across his forehead. An angiogram was recommended.

Don told the cardiologist his insurance had lapsed and he didn't have the cash to pay any large medical bills. If the angiogram was performed, it would take years for him to pay off the doctor's fee. The very next words out of the cardiologist's mouth were, "Well, I guess we don't have to rush into this. There is no reason why the angiogram can't wait." Don was sent home.

Don was determined to treat himself if the cardiologist wouldn't. He drank some water, took some potassium and magnesium supplements orally, and slowly returned to normal. Don has been *waiting* for his angiogram now for over a year and is doing just fine.

RACE

Race has been found to play a role in who gets cabbaged and who does not. Nationally the rate of having a cabbage surgery runs 27.1 per 10,000 whites per year, and only 7.6 per 10,000 blacks. Hospital admission rates for coronary artery disease for the two races are the same. The authors concluded that racial prejudice appears to influence cabbage surgery rates.[16]

There is another way of viewing this study. Black people with coronary artery disease are being spared a lot of unnecessary heart surgery because of racial discrimination.

BIASED RECOMMENDATIONS FOR CABBAGE SURGERY

Another issue involved in cabbage surgery is that the person who presents the sales pitch is the same person who makes a lot of money from the procedure. Self serving biases are hard at work.

The operation surgeon may charge between $3,000 and $6,000 for a cabbage. Multiply that by over 200 cabbages per year and it begins to add up to a respectable income. It is common for successful cabbage surgeons to bank over $1.5 million dollars a year. After overhead expenses this usually translates into a net income of over $1 million (before taxes). I don't believe any physician's services are worth that much.

Belief in their own technical abilities, a basic belief in the surgical approach to disease, and subconscious biases related to financial considerations cause heart surgeons to recommend cabbages more often than non-invasive cardiologists. It's wise to avoid situations where people who are trying to sell you something have a lot to gain from the sale. If possible, get a second, even a third opinion, from physicians who are not going to get a piece of the action from a surgical procedure.

A general surgeon in my community offered the observation. If he developed severe coronary artery disease and was going to have cabbage surgery, he would want his surgery done in a nearby city where cabbage surgery rates are high and surgeons have mastered technical aspects of the operation. However, he would never allow the decision to do surgery to be made in the city.

MEDIA CABBAGE SURGERY HYPE

The public have been given misleading information about cabbage surgery. The procedure has been glorified on television programs such as the long running medical series *Saint Elsewhere*. almost weekly Dr. Craig, the arrogant, fictional, chief of surgery, could be found taking care of a patient with coronary artery disease. Craig would egotistically say something like, "I am going to take this man down to surgery, do a bypass, and *save* his life."

The entire show followed a satirical theme about medicine. I suspect the public never realized Dr. Craig's comments may have been meant as a tongue in cheek joke. In real life a cabbage surgeon would be more likely to say (to his colleagues) something like, "Let's take this well insured guy down to surgery and *crack* his chest."

COW VEINS IN YOUR FUTURE?

The degree of religious devotion cabbage surgeons feel for their pet procedure is exemplified by the following business note from the *Wall Street Journal*. The price per share of Bio Vascular Inc. fell after the company disclosed some disappointing results from an overseas study.

The company treats cow veins with a proprietary technique after which they are sold for use as bypass grafts in humans. Such a bizarre step would only be necessary when a patient's own veins and internal mammary arteries are no longer available, usually because they have been used up during multiple cabbage surgeries.

The current research found the rate of closure of the cow vein bypass grafts was unacceptably high. But twelve months after bypass surgery, only one in seven grafts remained open.[17] Who knows what part of what animal researchers might dream of harvesting detour pipes from next.

THE SECOND OPINION CLINIC

Almost everyone except invasive cardiologists and cabbage surgeons agree too many invasive procedures are being performed. During the CASS study mentioned above a new concept emerged. It should be possible to accurately evaluate people with coronary artery disease and identify those who will do well without an invasive (surgical) procedure. Thomas B. Grayboys described such a program in 1987 in the *Journal of the American Medical Association*.[18]

A second opinion clinic was opened in Boston in 1982. The first published study from the clinic involved 88 patients who had been advised to have cabbage surgery elsewhere on the basis of ordinary angiograms. Some had been referred by insurance carriers who were hoping to get out of paying some large bills. Large insurance companies are well aware that about 85 percent of cabbages are unnecessary, and teach this fact during private seminars for their executives. However, they don't make this public.

Patients were evaluated with a history, physical, treadmill, and a non-invasive test of left ventricular function (pumping efficiency). If symptoms were not severe, and the left ventricle demonstrated normal function, the clinic advised against surgery in favor of medical therapy. This was the case in 84 percent of the patients. Sixty of these patients (81 percent) followed this advice and during the next two years none of them died.

Grayboys reported that abnormalities found in the (ordinary) angiogram had no value in trying to predict how well a patient would do in the future. He stated this diplomatically by saying that obstructions in arteries are not as important as how well the heart is *adjusting* to the obstructions. The function of the heart is to pump blood. If the pump is working normally, invasive procedures are not going to improve the pumping action. As the old saying goes, if something isn't broken, don't try to fix it.

Marks and colleagues at Duke University developed another method for evaluating heart patients using the treadmill test alone. A new scoring system was devised which incorporated the length of time a patient could stay on the treadmill, development of angina symptoms during the test, and severity of depression of the "ST" segment on the EKG.

People who were found to be in the low risk category were advised not to have angiograms. The average death rate in this group was only 0.25 percent per year over the next four years. In patients with scores indicating higher risk, the death rate was 5 percent per year.[19] This study demonstrated once again that heart patients can be identified whose risk of death is low. These patients do well without surgery, and they constitute the majority of people with the problem.

WHAT HAPPENS TO PEOPLE WHO REFUSE CABBAGE SURGERY?

It is generally reported that between 6 to 8 percent of people who are advised to have cabbage surgery turn down their golden opportunity. As you have seen, in the majority of cases surgery doesn't make a difference in how long somebody may live.

Whady Hueb and his associates on the medical faculty of the University of Sao Paul, Brazil, decided to follow a group of patients who refused cabbage surgery. A total of 2, 520 people were advised to have cabbage surgery on the basis of ordinary angiograms. Of these, 151 refused surgery and were managed medically for two to eight years (entrance into the study was staggered).

Among those with obstructions in one or two of their coronary arteries, the annual death rate in the follow up period was 0 percent. Among those individuals with obstructions in all three of their coronary arteries, the death rate was only 1.3 percent per year. Estimated overall chance of surviving eight years was 89 percent.[20]

It is common for patients who have had cabbage surgery five to ten years previously to credit the cabbage surgery for their longevity. Considering the data presented above, it is more likely they have done well because their left ventricles had not been damaged and the cabbage surgery had nothing to do with their good fortune.

HOW TO REFUSE SURGICAL PROCEDURES WITHOUT UPSETTING YOUR DOCTOR OR APPEARING TO CHALLENGE THE DOCTOR'S JUDGEMENT

As we have discussed, invasive procedures are done more often on patients who are male, white, and have good medical insurance. Therefore, if a surgical procedure has been advised and you don't want to go along with the recommenda-

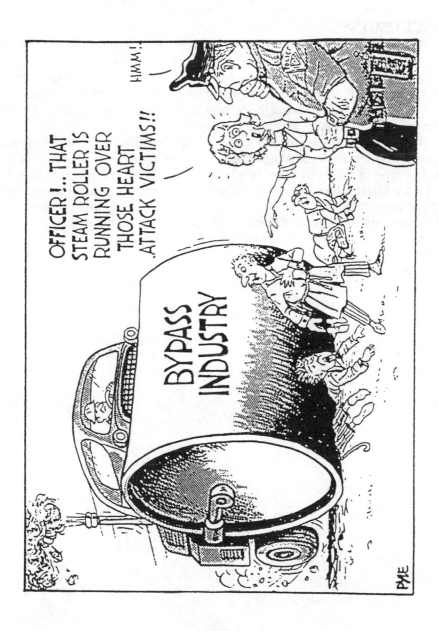

tion, consider doing this: Tell the surgeon your medical insurance just ran out, you are passing for white, you were a woman before your sex change operation, and you were recently exposed to the AIDS virus. At this point only the most aggressive of cabbage surgeons would continue to pressure you to sign an operative consent form.

CONCLUSIONS

The history of surgical approaches in the treatment of coronary artery disease is blackened by procedures which made no sense and didn't work. Cabbage surgery replaced these worthless procedures, and doesn't seem to be doing much better. Cabbage surgery has been found to relieve angina for a while in most patients who have symptoms, but not to extend life as most patients and doctors assume. It also carries with it a high rate of serious complications.

The cabbage surgery industry has developed a life of its own. Hospitals compete among themselves to attract cabbage surgeons and patients. Misconceptions about the value of these procedures are common among doctors and the public.

On the brighter side, several studies have confirmed it is possible to evaluate heart patients with non-invasive means and identify people who will do well with medical management alone. In the best of all worlds, this should become the wave of the future. But this will never occur as long as these crises situations remain under the control of people who are becoming rich by doing unnecessary surgical procedures.

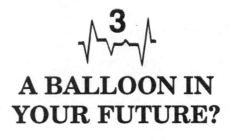

A BALLOON IN
YOUR FUTURE?

A SATIRICAL LOOK AT BALLOON ANGIOPLASTY

Soon it came to pass that a new breed of Western gun slinger appeared on the scene calling himself the *Invasive Cardiologist*. Like the hired gun, Paladin, he passed out business cards proclaiming, "HAVE CATHETER, WILL TRAVEL." At the first sign of trouble he would quick-draw out of his holster a five foot long tube and stick it into somebody's groin. On the end of the tube was a small latex balloon that appropriately looked like a condom.

The mere mention of the term *invasive cardiologist* sent chills up peoples' spines, and for good reason. In the past internists knew everything but did nothing. Suddenly they *knew* everything and *did* everything. These fellas were armed and dangerous.

The use of the term *invasive* in right-on. Somebody is going to be invaded and it isn't going to be the doctor. People who have seen these mavericks in action claim the slickest ones can stick a catheter into a groin and wind it around inside the body until it finds a wallet.

THE BALLOON PROCEDURE

The invasive cardiologist's claim to a lifestyle of the rich and famous is the balloon angioplasty. In this procedure a catheter is inserted up the aorta and threaded into the coronary arteries. The catheter can be passed into areas of obstruction in selected arteries.

At that point a balloon in its tip is inflated in an attempt to stretch the obstructed area. This must be done rapidly because blood flow through the artery is shut off while the balloon is inflated. If the balloon stays inflated too long it can cause a heart attack. The amazing thing is the stretched artery stays open for reasonable periods of time, at least in two out of three cases.

Performing this procedure sounds tricky, and it is. Care must be exercised in patient selection. The balloon can't be used in sections of arteries that are not straight. If arteries are too obstructed the catheter can't be passed. Some arteries are so hardened they can't be stretched. Many obstructions can't be reached with a balloon catheter.

39

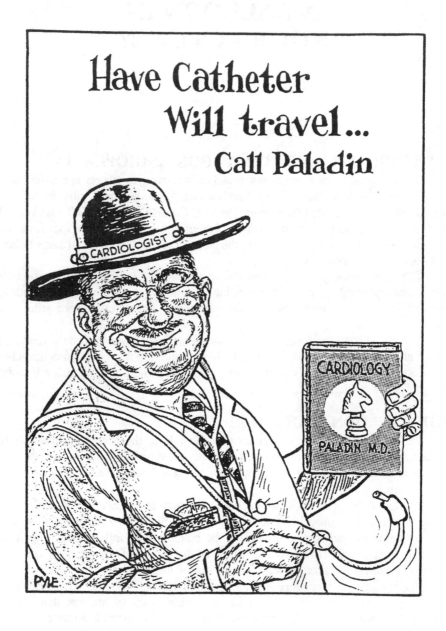

CABBAGE SURGEONS ATTACK
BALLOON PASSING CARDIOLOGISTS

When the balloon angioplasty first became available and spread across the land, cabbage surgeons felt threatened. They took up their scalpels and started a turf war.

Cardiologists who were learning to do balloon jobs were the enemy. These were the same people who had been referring patients to surgeons for cabbage surgery. Surgeons feared the wagon carrying the gold shipment was going to be cut off at the pass by a band of cardiologists wearing surgical masks. Heart surgeons' lifestyles were in serious jeopardy and it looked like the golden days might be coming to an end. They went public (within medicine, of course) claiming that the balloon job was an inadequately tested technique. This statement was accurate at the time.

The balloon job was promoted as a safer and far less expensive alternative to cabbage surgery. Stretching an artery with a balloon was going to correct plumbing problems without *cracking* the chest. Medical experts optimistically predicted that more heart cases would be handled successfully with balloons and the number of cabbage surgeries would go down. This would reduce health care costs. Such optimistic and far fetched expectations generally turn out to be laughable and there was no exception in this case. The greed factor had not been factored in.

Heart surgeons soon learned they had nothing to worry about. There was light at the end of the tunnel after all. As more and more balloon angioplastics were performed, the number of cabbages also increased. All vested interests soon slept better when they discovered the money pool available for surgical procedures on the heart resembled a bottomless pit. Medicine does not function according to supply and demand economics. If more physicians begin to divide up a medical pie, doctors can increase the size of the pie simply by recommending more procedures.

In 1990 invasive cardiologists performed about 285,000 balloon angioplasties and cardiac surgeons cracked 380,000 chests.[1] By 1996, according to the American Heart Association, the totals nearly doubled to 666,000 angioplasties and 598,00 coronary bypass procedures. That does not mean 1,264,000 different people were operated upon because many receive multiple procedures. It is not unusual to see patients who have had three or four balloon procedures followed by a cabbage, all within four or five months, and all failing to help. This may be good for doctors' incomes but it is not good for patients.

TRIAL BALLOONS

Innovators continue to look for ways to make the balloon angioplasty more successful. To prevent rapid re-obstruction, an inflatable metal *tent* has been developed which can be placed with the catheter, then popped open in the area of obstruction. This may appeal to Boy Scouts, but I wouldn't let any hungry *invasive cardiologist* set up a "tent" in one of my coronary arteries regardless what it may be called.

Other innovations are the hot laser, the cold laser, low speed drills, high speed drills, and tools that can scrape out and remove an area of obstructing material. The disease continues to be approached as a plumbing problem. I believe it would not be

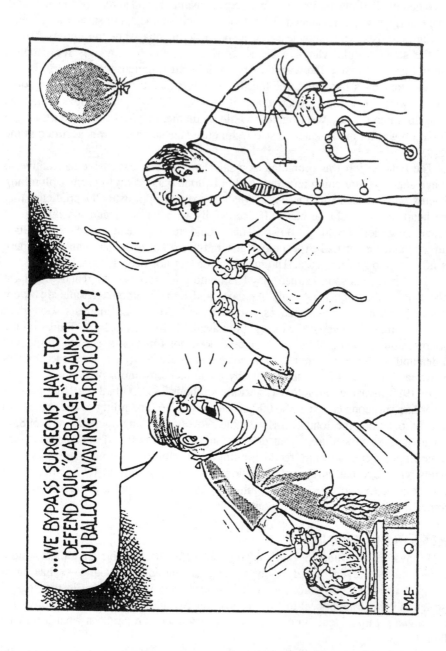

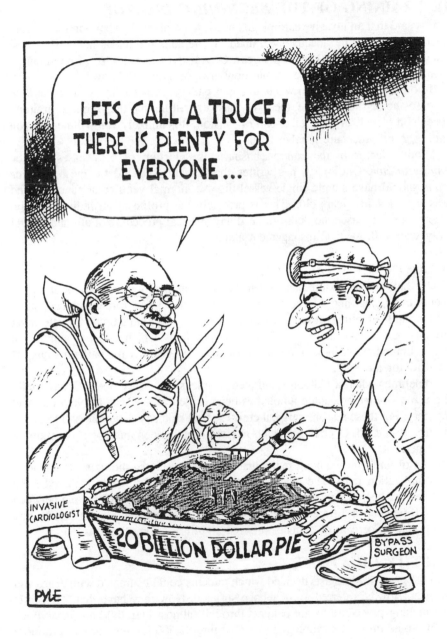

difficult to talk some cardiologist into injecting a little plumbing pipe cleaner into someone's coronary arteries (but not theirs). They have tried almost everything else.

THE TRAINING OF THE *BEGINNING DILATOR*

It is said that an invasive cardiologist needs to do about 150 balloon jobs before being considered to be adequately trained. To remain proficient he or she must continue to do at least 100 cases per year. Obviously it is not wise to be among a *beginning dilator's* first 150 cases, but how are you going to know?

If you ask some doc who wants to slip a balloon catheter into your groin how many cases he or she has done, the likely answer will be that the "required training has been completed" or some other sort of evasion. It is unlikely you will be told you are going to be procedure number five.

Another factor in the balloon business is selection of easy cases for the *beginning dilator*. One expert has written that patients selected for these *practice sessions* should have simple single-vessel disease, normal ventricular function, and be less than seventy years old.[2] This is precisely the profile of an individual with coronary artery disease who does not need any surgical procedure at all, and should do very well with medical management alone.[3]

BALLOON COMPLICATIONS

The balloon procedure has a substantial complication rate in addition to problems mentioned above. The coronary arteries don't like foreign objects stuck into them, and sometimes respond by going into spasm (contracting). Catheterizing a coronary artery can cause serious rhythm problems which can be fatal if not corrected immediately. In addition, a heart attack can occur if the balloon shuts off blood flow for too long.

Sometimes when a balloon is inflated it cracks the artery open. Occasionally during a *roto-rooter* procedure a hole has been drilled all the way through the wall of an artery. For these reasons surgical crews should be ready down the hall to swing into action if needed. Overall, the death rate with the balloon angioplasty is running about 2 percent.

Lack of uniformity among individual balloon passing cardiologists is apparent from complication rates. The worst statistics I have heard of were gathered from several smaller hospitals in Arizona. Death rates for balloon angioplasty ran between 5.5 and 20 percent in different hospitals. In the hospital with the highest death rate an additional 22 percent of patients suffered significant complications.

WEALTHY DILATORS

In the past, cardiologists decided which patients could be treated with drugs and which needed to be referred to a cabbage surgeon. Now they have their own little money making procedure to run patients through (almost literally) and from which to profit. Some invasive cardiologists are charging $2,500 for angiograms and more for balloon angioplasties. This is not small change for procedures which, respectively, are inaccurate and not proven to improve long term outcome.

Catheter passing cardiologists now can park their Rolls Royces next to those of cabbage surgeons in doctors' parking lots at hospitals. They can afford to join the *Medical Air Force* and fly their twin engine airplanes to favorite weekend retreats, all purchased with cash of course.

Dr. Robert Mendelsohn wrote in his book *Confessions of a Medical Heretic*, it is wise not to go to a doctor unless you absolutely must. It gives the doctor a chance to *intervene*. Invasive cardiologists have put a new spin on the word.

For years no studies existed comparing survival rates of heart attack victims treated medically or with balloon angioplasty. Studies finally did appear but conclusions are so mixed you can read them and draw any conclusion you wish according to your own biases.

A study in 1995 showed survival rates for a ten-year period were the same with invasive angioplasty as with a non-invasive clot dissolver. A 1996 study showed patients getting ballooned at hospitals performing many procedures had better survival rates than patients getting ballooned in smaller community hospitals where you and I would most likely be offered the procedure. Survival rates in the community hospitals were the same with angioplasty as with medical management alone.

In a 1999 study patients receiving a balloon angioplasty carried a 3 percent better chance of survival through a ten-year period than patients treated with the usual medical management.

What should we make of this? I certainly would not subject myself to a high-risk invasive procedure for a small difference in survival especially since I know of other effective and safe alternatives beyond being given a clot dissolver. In contrast, I asked a surgeon friend of mine what he would do given the same statistics and he said he would go for the balloon (a no-brainer).

STAMP OUT SILENT ISCHEMIA

Silent ischemia is a condition where some form of testing shows the heart muscle is not getting enough blood, even though the patient has no symptoms. Some academic cardiologists believe silent ischemia is a real thing, others say it is nothing more than a myth.

In efforts to promote sales of their electronic gadgets, medical equipment manufacturers are promoting the treatment of *silent ischemia*. Cardiologists are being encouraged to diagnose and treat the condition, thus producing many more candidates for balloon angioplasties.

Equipment manufacturers' advertisements in medical journals directed at invasive (catheter passing) cardiologists use marketing terms such as how to *penetrate* into new market areas, a highly appropriate use of the word. Invasive cardiologists need to learn state of the art marketing techniques because so many of them are being trained and competition is getting fierce. A surplus of invasive cardiologists means many have difficulty continuing to do the 100 cases per year needed to maintain proficiency in the procedure.

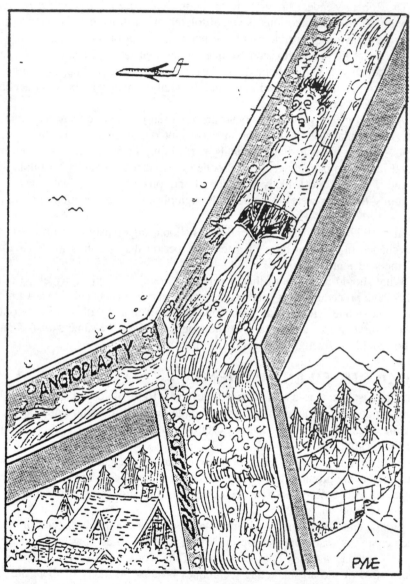

After an angiogram is performed it is difficult to turn off the medical mechinery that leads to either a balloon procedure or cabbage surgery.

THE SECOND OPINION CLINIC
AND ANGIOPLASTIES

Grayboys described evaluating 168 patients who were advised to have angiograms. After non-invasive out-patient evaluations, 80 percent were advised to not have the angiogram. Only 6 percent were advised to have the test right away. In the remaining patients a change in medical management was advised and the angiogram was deferred. Over the next 46 months the death rate for all 168 patients was only 1.1 percent per year.[4] This article received media attention and was presented on network evening news programs.

Patients in this study were not selected to represent the general population of heart patients. For this reason Grayboys revised his estimate of unnecessary angiograms down to a more conservative 50 percent. This was not enough to satisfy his critics. Some academic experts publicly attacked the study, saying these figures had to be too high because in *their* institutions they didn't do any unnecessary procedures. *Sure* they don't.

The only real reason to do an angiogram is to decide what to do during a surgical procedure. If, after non-invasive tests, a decision has been made to manage a patient medically, there is no reason to do an angiogram.

Once an angiogram has been done it is difficult to turn off the machinery that leads down a slippery slide into a cabbage or balloon job (see cartoon). If these types of second opinion evaluations were to become more routine, the majority of cabbages and angioplasties could be prevented. This would truly be a worthwhile form of preventive medicine. It also reminds me of two studies that showed that when doctors went on strike (in Israel and Los Angeles) death rates fell.

I am reminded of a invasive procedure a friend of mine had recently. This 58 year old doctor went to his cardiologist for a routine physical examination. Along with some lab tests a treadmill was ordered which showed a minor abnormality.

The cardiologist responded to this by recommending an angiogram (of ordinary pedigree). A small area of obstruction was found in one artery. My friend was told it would be a simple procedure to stick a balloon in there and stretch this obstruction to improve blood flow. This was carried out without complications.

By any standard this was an unnecessary procedure. The fact that the procedure was carried out by a friend demonstrates how brainwashed invasive cardiologists have become. Blind belief in the value of the procedure has reached religious proportions.

AN ASPIRIN A DAY KEEPS THE CATHETER AWAY

A revealing study was reported by Dr. Eugene Braunwald, professor of medicine at Harvard Medical School. Several hundreds of thousands of patients with stable angina from more than 40 hospitals were randomly divided into four groups and treated with either aspirin, nitroglycerin, a calcium channel blocking drug, or angioplasty. At the end of several years death rates were compared.

Death rates were fairly similar in all four of the groups, but the aspirin group had the lowest rate of death. The authors concluded that patients with stable angina

(angina that goes away or can be relieved with medicines) can be safely treated in their local community hospitals and don't need to be referred to larger facilities for invasive testing (angiograms) and treatment (balloons and cabbages).

BE CAREFUL

When confronted with an invasive cardiologist or cabbage surgeon, be on guard. Very likely a surgical procedure will be advised. Remember, if a craftsman's only tool is a hammer, every problem begins to look like a nail.

Heart disease victims should insist on having either an echocardiogram or nuclear medicine isotope scan to determine the *ejection fraction*, a measurement of how well the left ventricle is functioning as a pump. If the left ventricle is able to pump blood normally, then there is no evidence a cabbage or balloon procedure is going to improve chances of survival.

CONCLUSIONS

The balloon angioplasty has become a very popular procedure in the past 15 years. This has occurred despite the fact that no long term survival studies have been conducted. In professor Gbraunwald's most recent study, patients with coronary artery disease did just as well taking an aspirin a day as having a balloon job. Until any proof appears that people do better after being ballooned, it is wise to avoid having an invasive cardiologist *quick draw* his catheter on you.

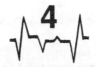

4

WHO BENEFITS FROM CABBAGE AND BALLOON PROCEDURES?

I got the bill for my surgery. Now I know why those doctors were wearing masks.

James H. Boren

Cabbage surgery and balloon procedures are prevalent, but they don't accomplish much and cost an arm and a leg. Such an illogical situation can persist only in a system where powerful vested interests benefit from the procedures. Some groups prospering from the procedures are obvious. Others are more obscure.

CABBAGE SURGEONS

Cabbage surgeons are the most obvious beneficiaries. A truly happy cabbage surgeon with a strong referral base may do as many as four to six cabbages a day. His surgical team may be busy enough to book two operating rooms at once. The cabbage surgeon may hire younger surgeons by the hour to perform the more mundane parts of the procedure, such as the *harvesting* of leg veins, opening the breast bone with a power saw, and closing the chest.

I am not kidding about the saw. The power tool looks like an ordinary jig saw with a protective tip to protect deeper structures. The breast bone is cut starting from the lower end and the entire procedure takes about as long as it takes to say zip, zip, zip, zip.

After the chest is open and the veins are laid out and oriented in the proper direction (they have one way valves and have occasionally been implanted in the wrong direction) the prima donna makes his grand entrance. The heart surgeon connects the patient to the heart lung machine, sews in from one to six individual bypass grafts, disconnects the heart lung machine, and stimulates the heart to begin beating again. This may take as little as 45 minutes. Then the surgeon is out of there and on to the next room, leaving assistants to do the *scut work* (sewing the chest wall back together, moving the patient to the recovery room, writing post-op orders).

After young heart surgeons get into private practice and see their incomes beginning to soar, some feel guilty about making so much money. Sixty years ago doctors frequently worked for nothing, a dollar per office visit, or accepted chickens and other live animals in exchange for their services. Now it is check, cash, plastic, or insurance.

The old docs may not have had many effective tools to work with, but they knew how to sit at the bedside, hold your hand and offer emotional support. Greed levels ran low. Doctors expected to work hard and live comfortable lives. They did not expect to join the ranks of the super rich.

Physicians' incomes began to rise rapidly during the 1970s. This became noticeable in the idle chatter surgeons carried on during dull surgical procedures. We used to talk about our families, interesting cases, and sex lives of stewardesses we had seen in the office (minus names). As large amounts of cash began to flood in the subject matter became dominated by the new problems of what to do with all the money.

Our vocabularies increased. We began to use words previously foreign to us such as puts, calls, selling short, long term capital gains, tax shelters, vesting, and 501Ks. We talked about who had made money in some shrewd deal, or who had lost money in some strange oil drilling investment some creep had talked him into.

Most highly paid physicians seemed to adjust quickly to the good economic times, soon developing an attitude that they must be worth every penny of what they are making. Why else would this be happening to them? Must be their good karma.

THE MAKING OF A CABBAGE SURGEON

I once knew a chest surgeon who wanted to move up in status and become a cabbage surgeon. Unfortunately, Dr. X took his training before bypass surgery fellowships had become available. A friend joked that when this fellow graduated from medical school he must have decided to specialize in diseases of the rich.

One of his most satisfied patients was a lady who qualified to be called *super rich*. After Dr. X had done some tinkering around inside of her chest she had done well and thought her doctor walked on water. Dr. X was already aware he could walk on water. But he found he could pull this stunt off only on days he had done surgery. Possibly if he became a cabbage surgeon he would be able to walk on water any time he wished.

The rich patient asked what he might like as a gift, telling him he could have anything his heart desired. Never dreaming his wish might come true, Dr. X asked if she would consider donating a heart lung machine to the hospital for research. A few weeks later a truck arrived and off-loaded the $100,000 machine.

Dr. X set up an animal laboratory in the basement of the hospital where he practiced doing bypasses on healthy dogs. In retrospect, it was most appropriate for a future bypass surgeon to practice on subjects who didn't need surgery. Most of his future patients wouldn't need the surgery either. After several months, the hospital allowed him to begin doing cabbages on humans.

It didn't pay to be one of the first patients in Dr. X's new program because, as usual, his death rate started off quite high. Before long the bypass grafts leaked less often and deaths became more infrequent, eventually declining to acceptable levels.

Dr. X couldn't have timed his new venture better. Americans had fallen in love with cabbage surgery. It was just *so* high tech. In many social circles if you didn't have a recent scar down the middle of your chest you were considered to be boring at cocktail parties.

Dr. X's practice mushroomed. Before long, he was head of a busy four-man cabbage surgery practice. His toys escalated in value as well. Soon he was able to trade in his Porsche for a new Rolls Royce. He bought a new twin Beech, joined the local chapter of the *Medical Air Force*, and flew to weekend destinations in formation with other successful physicians. He even told us what a good *investment* he had made in the Rolls, not realizing how badly he was conning himself.

I was not concerned about these events at the time. If a doctor friend of mine hit the jackpot I was happy. Maybe uterine transplants would become the next fad and one day a humble gynecologist also might be able to fly with the *Medical Air Force*.

Then something happened that soured my opinion of Dr. X. Several of us were in the surgeons' dressing room changing clothes when he decided to unload some emotional garbage that had been irritating him.

His brother owned a fruit ranch and was having a problem with the state department of agriculture. The state had passed regulations mandating that ranchers had to provide more outhouses for migrant farm workers, the number to be decided on a head count.

Dr. X's brother resented this governmental intrusion into his affairs. Both Dr. X and his brother felt that the state had no right to dictate how many outhouses the migrant could use. Expenditures of supplying outhouses would come directly out of the ranch's bottom line. It was bad enough that ranchers had to provide the lowly migrant workers with small shacks (with no running water) so they could have a roof over their heads at night. Wealthy Dr. X's lack of compassion left a permanent impression one me.

KING OF CABBAGE

Julian Whitaker, M.D., tells of the financial opportunities of a cabbage surgeon who was a salaried faculty member of Emory University Medical School in Atlanta. A professor in some less glamorous specialty discovered the school was paying the cabbage surgeon $500,000 a year. This was more than seven times the income of any other member of the medical faculty at the time. The professor asked the dean of the school for an explanation.

The situation really was very simple. The school had to pay the man a high salary to keep him on the faculty. If the cabbage surgeon had chosen to leave the university and enter private practice, he could easily have netted $1.5 million a year because of his prestige and referral base.

Not all cabbage surgeons make that kind of money. In the *dark side* of medicine active competition exists between heart surgeon groups and a form of marketing greases referrals from other physicians, especially cardiologists. Therefore, though 15 percent of cabbage surgeons net over $600,000 per year (1998 *Medical Economics* survey) many must limp along almost on food stamps netting only $200,000 or $300,000 a year.

Why did the medical school want to keep him on the payroll so desperately? Medical schools run hospitals. Therefore, in addition to educating future doctors, they must worry about mundane things such as cash flows, profits and losses. Hospitals that do cabbage surgery make money. A marketing expert in the health care field reported that hospitals made an average net profit of $4,049 per bypass patient in 1988[1]

ASSISTANT CABBAGE SURGEONS

Cabbage surgeons need another surgeon to assist during the procedure. The fictional Ben Casey may have done brain surgery all by himself every week on television, but it doesn't work that way in real life.

Surgeons who assist in surgery generally bill for an amount equal to 20 percent of the operating surgeon's fee. Twenty percent of the current average surgeon's fee of $5,474 (*Medical Economics*, 1998) is not bad pay for a couple of hours work. The icing on the cake is that the assistant isn't slowed down by being forced to talk with the patient and hearing of every old ache and pain as well as updates on bowel function of the day. The first and last time the assistant surgeon sees the victim is in the operating room after he or she has been zonked by the anesthetic.

Most of the time surgical assistants are themselves cabbage surgeons who share an office with the operating cabbage physician. They help each other primarily because of their expertise, but they also appreciate the extra cash, which to them must seem like loose change.

ANESTHESIOLOGISTS

Anesthesiologists benefit from bypass surgery. In medical slang anesthesiologists are called gas passers. Anesthesiologists use measured amounts of poisons to put surgical patients to sleep and, hopefully, wake them up. They bill patients by the hour. Each cabbage case may take about two to three hours of their time. They have nothing to do with the decision to do surgery, but you don't hear any of them making waves by complaining about unnecessary surgery. To do so would jeopardize their standing in the anesthesia department and their livelihoods.

I once felt sorry for anesthesiologists because they were forced to watch inept surgeons botch surgical procedures and say nothing. I don't feel so sorry for them any more. Now, anesthesiologists can afford to drive Rolls Royces and fly their own twin engine private airplanes in the *Medical Air Force*.

CARDIOLOGISTS

Cardiologists benefit. A cardiologist must be present during bypass surgery to handle medical emergencies that may arise. Sometimes the patient's heart may go into an abnormal rhythm when surgeons zap it to start beating again when the heart lung machine has been disconnected.

When all is going well the cardiologist has a lot of free time on his hands. He may just stand around telling jokes. Though he is enjoying himself and doing nothing, his meter is still ticking at a rate of $200 per hour and up.

Then there is the other breed of cardiologist, the balloon passer. These cardiologists have done quite well for themselves during the past decade. Balloon procedures were rare before 1980. In 1990 there were 280,000 balloon procedures in the United States. Balloon passing cardiologists are well qualified to fly in the *Medical Air Force*.

OTHER HOSPITAL PERSONNEL BENEFIT

Many hospital employees derive their incomes form surgical procedures on the heart. Many highly trained people must be present in the operating room during bypass surgery. There are layers and layers of surgical nurses and technicians. Ten or more highly trained employees may be in the operating room at one time.

Cabbage surgery and balloon procedures support extra staff people in post-operative areas during recuperation. Later, dietitians arrive to give heart patients worthless advise such as following the diet of the American Heart Association. Exercise specialists enter the picture later during rehabilitation.

EQUIPMENT MANUFACTURERS

Cabbage surgery requires an operating room large enough to hold all of the required equipment. The heart lung machine itself is large and its operation requires a specially trained technician. All types of monitors are involved, such as EKG machines, blood gas monitors, a cardiac output monitor, and a central venous pressure monitor, in addition to multiple instrument trays. The list goes on and on.

Other manufacturers of surgical supplies get cut in for a piece of the action. These include producers of anesthetic gases, sutures, instruments, retractors, tubing, dressings, skin preps, sponges, drapes, lights, operating tables. The list is enormous, and the items are not cheap.

If you have the opportunity and a strong heart study an itemized hospital bill for surgery. You may not be able to understand most of the bill because it will be in a foreign language, a medical jargon most people will instantly associate with Greek. You may not be able to decipher the items listed, but their dollar values are always crystal clear.

It is no joke that if some item is suddenly recognized to have a medical application, someone will say, *"Oh my God, this is a piece of medical equipment!"* That revelation alone is enough to increase its price many fold. According to a recent news report, one cabbage patient was billed $10 for a Band-Aid.

DRUG COMPANIES

In every itemized bill for bypass surgery you will probably find thousands of dollars of charges for drugs used during the hospital stay. And this has nothing to do with various medications that will be advised for home use after the patient is discharged. Many will be prescribed for lifetime use.

INSURANCE COMPANIES

Top level executives can benefit from bypass surgery. The more money an insurance company is handling the more its executives can justify paying themselves in salaries and perks. If the frequency of bypass surgeries and balloon procedures fell to reasonable levels, probably 5 to 10 percent of current numbers, billions of dollars less would pass through private insurance companies. Executives might be forced to do the unthinkable and take pay cuts.

In the past, insurance companies did not have any incentive to reduce health care costs. They protected their profits and avoided being surprised by some new expensive treatment they did not anticipate. Things are changing. Large corporations are beginning to limit how much they will pay for health care benefits for their workers. This will result in reduced coverage so more medical cost will be dumped back on the individual consumer.

Reductions in coverage are going to become more prevalent in self-insured plans. A recent U.S. Supreme Court Decision allowed companies with self-insured plans to reduce maximum benefits workers may receive, in this case even after the employee had become ill. How this will ripple back through the health care system and Congress is unknown.

HOSPITALS BENEFIT

Hospitals that do cabbage surgery and balloon procedures usually make money, a lot of money. They compete with other hospitals to attract bypass surgeons, frequently offering to buy any and all of the equipment and fancy gadgets the cabbage surgeons' little hearts may desire. If a hospital can lure a bypass surgery team away form a competing hospital, a major financial coup has been pulled off that translates into millions of dollars of additional profit per year.

The obvious motivation is money. As mentioned above, American hospitals averaged a net profit of over $4,000 for each bypass surgery performed in 1988. However, the opportunity exists for hospitals to milk the system for a lot more than that.

Consumer Reports described an example of the crazy way hospitals bill for bypass surgery. The state of Pennsylvania conducted a survey of hospital charges for cabbage surgery, then made the results public. One hospital in Erie was found to be charging $14,000 more for a heart bypass operation than a local competing hospital. The high flying hospital reacted to the public report by dropping its charges by $10,000.[2]

VESTED INTERESTS

With all the people involved in balloon and cabbage procedures, this creates a long list of vested interests. I believe the term, *medical-industrial-pharmaceutical-complex* is well justified. This is not an equitable, reasonable system. A small minority of patients may benefit from surgical procedures directed at their coronary artery disease, yet every year tens of billions of dollars are spent on unnecessary procedures.

This is but one example of the danger of leaving health care decisions in the hands of doctors. Foxes should not be allowed to guard chicken houses. Physicians are not immune from encouraging and over-utilizing procedures that benefit themselves, even if they must first delude themselves into justifying their actions.

PATIENTS BENEFIT THE LEAST

In some cases cabbage surgery or a balloon procedure is performed because of chest pain that can't be relieved with rest or through the application of other approaches. Most experts believe this may be a reasonable indication for surgery at this time. It may not make much sense in the future if more doctors would begin to apply other helpful approaches which are not taught in medical schools (described later).

Most patients who receive cabbage surgery or a balloon stretching procedure don't have intractable pain. They have hearts that function (pump) normally and don't need any surgery. According to second opinion studies and other sources, as many as 85 percent of patients with heart problems will do just fine without being cracked open or ballooned.

Usually patients who are most likely to die or have a serious complication are not offered a chance to lie down on the operating table and have a procedure. These are the patients that would cause death rates for heart surgeries to go up. Surgeons and hospitals don't want to see their death rates from these procedures rise too high. This may upset state inspectors who keep tabs on matters such as this (but don't make the statistics public).

SUMMARY

As Harvard professor Braunwald predicted, a financial empire has developed around surgical procedures on the heart. With so many powerful vested interests involved, it will be difficult to change how American doctors treat patients with coronary artery disease. No one who is currently gaining from the system has any incentive to try to stop the unnecessary costs and suffering.

5

CHOLESTEROL-PHOBIA

There is always an easy solution to every problem...neat, plausible and wrong.

H.L. Mencken

A true believer in the cholesterol theory must be willing to genuflex before the following statements with a religious fervor:

1. Eating cholesterol and saturated fats raises the blood cholesterol level.
2. Elevated blood levels of cholesterol cause fatty deposits to form in our arteries.
3. Eating less saturated fat and cholesterol will cause blood levels of cholesterol to go down.
4. Lowering blood cholesterol levels (by any means) will reduce the risk of dying.

There is just one simple problem with these assumptions. They are all wrong.

The cholesterol theory came to life as part of an effort to try to understand why people develop coronary artery disease. The cholesterol connection was a logical concept to pursue. In the early stages it looked very promising.

The material that obstructs artery walls visually resembled common fatty foods such as butter, lard, and beef tallow. Fatty obstructions in arterial walls were found to contain fibrin, calcium, cholesterol, and several other fatty materials. Heart attacks were found to be more common in countries where people eat more fats. Feeding high fat diets to animals produced fatty deposits in their coronary arteries.

The circumstantial evidence was impressive and led experts to conclude that eating a diet high in fats and cholesterol must cause coronary artery disease in humans. Unfortunately, efforts to prove the cholesterol theory have failed. In addition, experts have chosen to ignore all exceptions to the theory in their efforts to keep the hypothesis intact.

The cholesterol theory is not compatible with the history of coronary artery disease. Dietary consumption of fats and cholesterol does not effect blood levels of cholesterol significantly in the vast majority of people. Many people with high blood

56

cholesterols never experience coronary artery disease. People with low blood cholesterols can and do develop coronary artery disease. About one-third of people who have a heart attack have a blood cholesterol level that is well within the range accepted as normal. Attempts to lower death rates from coronary artery disease with the American Heart Association diet have consistently failed. In addition, when drugs are given to try to lower blood cholesterol, overall death rates have gone *up*, not down as anticipated.

After forty years of research, promoters are still trying to sell the theory, but they can't demonstrate that their efforts have had any effect on the disease. Coronary artery disease was the leading cause of death in 1950 and it remains entrenched in first place today.

A BRIEF HISTORY OF CORONARY ARTERY DISEASE

Americans have always eaten a high fat diet. This fact has led backers of the cholesterol theory to conclude that we always must have suffered from heart attacks as well. Believers in the cholesterol theory point out that archaeologists found hardening of the arteries (arteriosclerosis) in 3,000 year old Egyptian mummies. But this does not prove either that arteriosclerosis was common among Egyptians or that it led to heart attacks.

It is more likely that findings in mummies of members of the ruling class of ancient Egypt are not representative of the majority of people who lived at that time. Upper class Egyptians were known to have followed different diets and lifestyles than their underlings. For example, they satisfied their cravings for sweets by sending unprotected slaves to gather honey. This led to the development of tooth decay that was not found in bodies of poor people.

IT ALL STARTED IN 1878

The first published case of a proven heart attack appeared in a British medical journal in 1878, a little over 100 years ago. The patient had crushing chest pain, collapsed and died. At autopsy an area of fatty necrosis (dead muscle) was found in the heart. There may have been a few other heart attacks before this, but Adam Hammer gets the credit for writing the first report.[1] A historical perspective is needed to appreciate the importance of this report.

Interest in the newly developing medical sciences was running high in Europe between 1830 and 1880. Physicians discovered and named most of our diseases during that time. The most famous pathologists of all time were busy cutting up and examining as many bodies as they could. In some parts of Austria autopsies were performed automatically by royal decree. Pathologists performed tens of thousands of autopsies during a period of about fifty years. However, there is no record of a single case of a heart attack until 1878. Also missing are descriptive reports of people suffering chest pains and dropping dead in the street, a common occurrence now.

American medical experts don't want to accept this fact, and hyperinflated egos of doctors also get in the way of reason. Modern doctors prefer to assume that old fashioned doctors (meaning less well trained than now) did see patients with heart attacks, but were too dumb to recognize them. In defense of the old, well meaning, but stupid doctors, it is emphasized that they didn't have modern high tech tools with which to make an accurate diagnosis (i.e., EKG machines).

Samuel Levine, professor of medicine at Harvard University during the 1950s, promoted this concept. Levine wrote, "It is difficult to understand how the great clinicians of the past, many of whom performed many postmortem (autopsy) examinations, could have overlooked this problem, especially when it is appreciated that the recognition of coronary thrombosis (heart attack) developed from a purely clinical study of patients without the use of any elaborate procedures or laboratory methods that characterize the modern era of medicine."[2] Levine may have written like a lawyer, but his point is clear.

OBSERVATIONS OF PAUL DUDLEY WHITE

Paul Dudley White founded the specialty of cardiology and became a public figure when he served as physician to President Eisenhower during Ike's in-office heart attack. White graduated from medical school in 1910. He later wrote that as a young man he had an interest in the heart attack problem and had been looking for such cases after reading about them in the European literature.

White saw his first heart attack patient in 1921 after he had been in practice for eleven years. It was his opinion that heart attacks were rare to absent before that time.[3] When he was a much older man a reporter asked for his opinion about the cholesterol theory. White said he couldn't support the theory because he knew it didn't fit the history of the disease.

Europeans began to code the heart attack as a separate cause of death in 1930. The United States did not begin to record it separately until 1950. Before that time heart attack deaths were lumped with deaths from diseases of the kidneys, other heart diseases of all types, and high blood pressure.

TABLE 1
Death Rates from Coronary Artery Disease and Fat Consumption
in the United States, 1910-1990[4]

Year	Deaths/100,000	Total Fat	Saturated Fat	Cholesterol
1910	10	125 gm	50 gm	509 mg
1920	9	NA	NA	NA
1930	46	135	53	524
1940	134	133	53	493
1950	212	141	54	577
1960	274	143	55	578
1970	331	155	59	540
1980	249	158	58	500
1985	224	169	61	500
1990	194	NA	NA	NA

Death rates from 1910 to 1940 are from Seattle. Death rates from 1950 to 1990 are for the U.S. NA = not available.

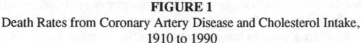

FIGURE 1
Death Rates from Coronary Artery Disease and Cholesterol Intake,
1910 to 1990

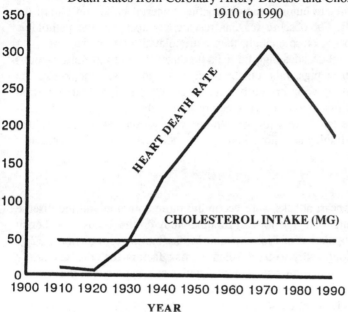

The death rate from coronary artery disease went up 3,010 percent between 1910 and 1970. During this time total fat consumption went up 25 percent, saturated fat 18 percent, and cholesterol up 8 percent. From 1970 to 1985 total fat consumption rose another 9 percent while the death rate from heart attacks fell by about one-third.

The most plausible reason why nobody coded the heart attack separately was because it was a rare event. However, some isolated localities began to code heart attacks separately before 1950. Death rates in King County (Seattle), Washington, and the U.S. from 1910 to 1990 are summarized in Table 1. Also shown is fat consumption for the United States.

The lack of a relationship between the death rate from coronary artery disease and saturated fat and cholesterol intake is best shown graphically as in Figure 1.

In the past forty years the death rate from coronary artery disease has behaved unpredictably. It rose from a rate of 212 per 100,000 population in 1950, to 331 per 100,000 in 1968. At that point the trend reversed itself and the rate had fallen to 194 per 100,000 by 1990.[5]

During those forty years fat consumption in the United States was almost constant. This is why people in the cholesterol camp have never tried to take credit for the decline in death rates since 1968. Most authorities give the credit to changes individuals have made in their diets and lifestyles, as well as to improvements in emergency care of heart attacks in coronary care units.[6]

THE BIRTH OF THE CHOLESTEROL THEORY

In 1911 Antishkow and Ignatowski independently published the results of animal feeding studies related to cholesterol. Vegetarian rabbits ate a high fat/high cholesterol diet for several months and their blood cholesterol levels rose dramatically.[7] At autopsy the arteries of their hearts were plugged up with a fatty/fibrinous material.

However, the obstructions in the rabbits' arteries did not resemble those seen in humans. In rabbits the obstructing materials were found to be sticking to the inner lining of the arterial wall. In humans the obstructing material builds up within the wall of the artery itself. For obscure reasons researchers accepted the pathologic findings in rabbits as being close enough, then extrapolated them to humans.

Over the next several decades high fat diets produced similar fatty obstructions in vegetarian pigs, guinea pigs, rats, chicken, pigeons and rhesus monkeys. The feeding experiment didn't work in carnivorous dogs. Obstructions did not form unless the thyroid was first removed. This demonstrated that carnivores, or omnivores including humans, are born with the chemistry to handle fat in the diet. Fat researchers ignored the finding and moved onward in their efforts to prove what they had come to believe.

FRAMINGHAM

By the late 1940s heart attacks were becoming more common and the disease finally attracted some attention. The longest running study on the disease was begun in 1948. Most of the population of Framingham, Massachusetts (population 5,127), volunteered for a life-long study to try to identify risk factors for coronary artery disease. Researchers examined all risk factors popular at the time. An association was found between high blood cholesterol levels and heart attacks, but the connection was weak and barely measurable.

Investigators chose not to publicize another association that was found in the Framingham study that ran contrary to the cholesterol theory. Dietary intake of cholesterol and fats did not influence blood cholesterol levels. Some people who ate large amounts of saturated animal fat and cholesterol had low blood cholesterol levels. Some people who ate small amounts of saturated fat and cholesterol had high blood cholesterol levels.

TECUMSEH

In Tecumseh, Michigan, 4,057 people volunteered for a similar study and the findings came out the same. People with high blood cholesterols had a slightly greater risk of having heart attacks. But, once again, dietary intake of cholesterol was not related to blood cholesterol levels the way researchers anticipated.[8]

INTERNAL FEED BACK LOOPS

Dietary fat intake has little effect on blood cholesterol levels in most people because of an internal feed-back system. The process functions in a manner similar to a thermostat controlling a furnace to maintain a constant temperature in a home.

For unknown reasons the body sets a blood cholesterol level it likes, then tries to keep it constant. If you eat more cholesterol, the body makes less. If you eat less, the body makes more. Only a small percentage of people find they can alter their blood cholesterols up or down by more than 5 percent by changing their intake of cholesterol and fat. Normally about 80 percent of cholesterol in the blood is made in the body, most of it in the liver.

In recent years television commercials have portrayed cholesterol as the nastiest of villains and fat as public enemy *number one*. In one commercial cholesterol was depicted as an overweight, short, greasy little man wearing a dirty gray sweat shirt with "CHOLESTEROL" printed across the from in big black letters.

Actually, cholesterol is an essential compound in the body. The body uses cholesterol as the basic building material for making vitamin D, sex hormones, cortisone, and other materials we can't live without. Normal brain tissue contains high concentrations of cholesterol.

THE HEART ASSOCIATION ACCEPTS
THE CHOLESTEROL THEORY

With nothing more to go on than these weak associations, the American Heart Association decided eating fats and cholesterol caused heart attacks. Spokespeople began to promote the theory as if they were religious evangelists spreading a new gospel throughout the land. This irrational action stirred academic debate.

Dr. Alfred E. Harper, professor of biochemistry and nutritional sciences at the University of Wisconsin, and past president of the Food and Nutrition Board, pointed out exceptions to the theory in several countries. In Israel, Chile, and a few other low-cholesterol consumption countries, the incidence of coronary artery disease was high. In Scandinavian countries, fat consumption dropped while the incidence of the disease went up. As the consumption of animal fat in Switzerland increased, its rate of coronary artery disease went down.[9] Thus, the connection between dietary fats, cholesterol, and heart attacks was anything but consistent. This was a far different story than the American Heart Association was telling us and continues to preach.

THE *INTERVENTION* TRIALS

Lipid (fat) researchers ignored all exceptions and tried harder and harder to prove the validity of their theory. Many diet manipulation studies were begun, including two large *intervention* trials. An intervention trial is a study in which a treatment approach is used in one group of people to see if it will help prevent or treat a disease. Results are compared with a second group of untreated people (the control group).

MR. FIT

Results form the MRFIT (Multiple Risk Factor Intervention Trial) study were released in 1982. The study recruited 12,866 high risk men between the ages of 35 and 57. Researchers randomly divided the men into two groups.

One group went on a program to reduce the commonly accepted risk factors. This included a program to stop smoking, a low fat/low cholesterol diet, and treating high blood pressure with drugs. The other group ate an average American diet and received routine medical care. The study ran for seven years and cost American taxpayers $150,000,000.

When the investigation was completed, lipid researchers had to be disappointed. The heart attack death rate in the treatment group was slightly lower than in the control group. However, the overall death rate was higher in the treatment group because of an increase in cancer deaths.[10] Only the favorable results were publicized. Failure to report studies honestly soon became the standard modus operandi for fat researchers.

LIPIDS RESEARCH CLINICS STUDY

The second large intervention trial was the Lipids Research Clinics Study.[11] In this study the effects of a cholesterol-lowering drug, colestyramine, were compared to a placebo (an inactive material). A screening process identified 3,810 high risk men who had cholesterols higher than 95 percent of the population. Researchers divided the randomly men into two groups.

Both groups went to the low fat diet of the American Heat Association. One group took the drug colestyramine in addition to following the diet. There were 19 percent fewer heart attack deaths in the drug group than in the control group.

From this data it was calculated that for every 1 percent drop in blood cholesterol, the risk of death from a heart attack went down by 2 percent. This was the first study that produced *any* results supportive of the cholesterol theory. These numbers were highly publicized and have become imprinted on the floppy discs in physicians' brains.

Backers of the fat hypotheses proclaimed they had at long last proven the cholesterol theory. Other researchers remained unconvinced. Some pointed out it was inappropriate to express the changes as percentages. A 10 percent drop in serum cholesterol from 400 to 360 mg/dl would probably produce greater benefits than a 10 percent drop from 200 to 180 mg/dl.

Also, if a blood cholesterol level fell by 51 percent or more, then the risk of having a heart attack could go down by more than 100 percent, a mathematical impossibility. Others pointed out these findings came from a group of high risk men and it was inappropriate to apply them to the general population. But this was exactly what was being done and continues to be done to this day.

The most important criticism involved information that was not publicized about death rates. There were three times as many deaths from suicide, homicide and trauma in the drug treatment group as among controls. When those deaths were included in the analysis, there was no improvement in overall death rates in the drug treatment group. Once again, researchers had reported results in a misleading way.

These results have been regurgitated to this day and are used as indefensible ways. When a treatment lowers blood cholesterol a few points, the authors use these numbers to extrapolate how many lives might be saved if the method was applied to the masses.

THE CONSENSUS DEVELOPMENT CONFERENCE

Armed with results from the positive side of this single study, lipid scientists were eager to take the next step, the establishment of a set of dietary recommendations for the entire population of the United States. To facilitate this effort a new disease had to be invented they called it *hypercholesterolemia*, which means a blood level above a certain arbitrary level selected by fat researchers. This new *disease* has no connection to the overall health of an individual.

The National Heart, Lung and Blood Institute of the National Institutes of Health convened the Consensus Development Conference in Bethesda, Maryland, in December, 1984. A panel of 14 cholesterol experts heard papers and reviews covering more than 30 years of research. Planners scheduled less than three days for the conference.

Most of the speakers were long time believers in the cholesterol theory. Speakers presented many aspects of years of research, almost all of it in support of the cholesterol theory.

Dr. Richard Peto, from Oxford University in England, drew the difficult task of explaining why all of the attempts to lower blood cholesterol had failed to lower overall death rates. His explanation was that there had "already been 15 or 20 trials, but in every one something *ridiculous* happened."[12]

This means efforts to reduce overall death rates with the American Heart Association's diet failed in every study. It was difficult to document anything more than a weak association between dietary cholesterol intake and coronary artery disease in one study out of 20. Even in that study overall death rates did not go down. This did not support the cholesterol theory as being a leading risk factor for the disease. A logical individual would think that cholesterol researchers should have begun to wake up and discover that their favorite risk factor was noting more than a paper tiger. This did not happen.

Many researchers present at the meeting were more cautious. Some pointed out there were problems with the cholesterol studies and many facets of coronary artery disease remained unknown. They took the position it was unwise to rush to issue national dietary guidelines on the evidence available. Their objections were ignored.

At the end of the second day the chairperson made an announcement that shocked many attendees. "It has been established beyond a reasonable doubt that lowering elevated blood cholesterol levels will reduce the risk of heart attack deaths due to coronary artery disease." As mentioned above, among the 20 studies conducted, only the Lipids Research Clinics Study showed this relationship, and in that case there was no overall reduction in death rates because of an increase in deaths from other causes.

The panel decided a *consensus* existed and a national cholesterol education program was the next logical step to take. That was not all. Printed copies of the plan were scheduled to be distributed at 8:30 the next morning and the program would be announced to the public at a press conference three hours later. The hidden agenda of the meeting was finally revealed. Promoters of the cholesterol theory must have planned these steps weeks to months before the meeting took place.[13] This was really no *consensus development meeting* at all.

This is one of the most bizarre actions ever taken in medicine. Medicine has a centuries old pattern of not accepting revolutionary new breakthroughs until several decades have passed. In many cases this means the opposition must die off. In this case the opposite occurred. There was a rush to judgment based on bias and belief. Caution was thrown to the wind.

E.H. Ahrens, of Rockefeller University, pointed out problems with this rush to judgment. In 20 studies researchers had tried to prove a reduction in dietary fat and cholesterol would reduce coronary artery disease events. Only one study showed any association in this direction at all and that is what would be expected by chance alone. If the scientific method had been applied the unusual study would be thrown out, not the nineteen that were consistent.

Ahrens was very candid and wrote, "I would have been content with the consensus statement if it had confined itself to what we do know and what we do not. It promises benefits without giving the evidence to back up that promise. By failing to emphasize what we do not know, the statement sweeps these weaknesses in our evidence under the rug, as if they were trivial. I have disagreed with that position."[14]

CROSS CULTURAL PATTERNS OF CORONARY ARTERY DISEASE

A comparison of heart attack death rates in other countries creates more problems for the cholesterol theory. Many groups of people in the world have remained free of the disease, at least in the past. Some drastic exceptions to the theory exist such as groups that consumed diets that were very high in saturated fats, yet ran low blood cholesterols and had no heart attacks.

Some examples of populations discovered to have no heart attacks were the following:

- Tribal Africans[15]
- The Masai of East Africa[16]
- Africans in Western Transvaal[17]
- Natives of Degestan, Russian Caucasus[19]
- Elderly Ugandans[20]
- Natives of the Republic of Zaire[21]
- Semi-isolated people of the Loetschental Valley of Switzerland[22]
- Yemenites in the holy land.[23]
- Many more areas are reviewed in another article[24]

This is not a complete list. It is representative of the general finding of the almost total absence of coronary artery disease in primitive lifestyles people. Some of these studies were based on autopsy findings in people who were over sixty.

THE MASAI

Western medical experts have thoroughly studied the Masai tribe in Africa. The Masai live in East Kenya and Northern Tanzania and are a nomadic people who number over 100,000. They heard cattle, goats, and sheep, and don't intermarry with other tribes. Most of their diet consists of fresh, raw cow's milk. Adults consume up to five liters of milk a day.

Masai frequently mix milk with blood collected from their cattle. About 66 percent of calories in the diet are in the form of saturated fat. Masai run cholesterols of only 135 mg/dl and don't have heart attacks as long as they live their traditional lifestyle away from civilization.

American cholesterol researchers traveled to Kenya and studied the Masai. Dietary cholesterol intake was manipulated in volunteers. When fed 2,000 mg a day of cholesterol (one egg yolk contains about 300 mg) blood cholesterols averaged 135 mg/dl. When fed no cholesterol at all blood cholesterol levels stayed the same. About all the researchers could say about this was that people in the Masai tribe must have perfect internal feed back mechanisms for cholesterol. This was assumed to be related to a protective hereditary trait.[25]

DO HIGH BLOOD LEVELS OF CHOLESTEROL PREDICT HEART ATTACKS?

In preparation for the MRFIT study, researchers screened 356,222 men between the ages of 35 and 57. All men had blood cholesterol drawn and were followed for six years. The most positive connections between blood cholesterol levels and heart attacks were in the group aged 55 to 57.

In men with cholesterol levels below 180 mg/dl the coronary artery disease death rate was 8.3 per 1,000. In men with cholesterols over 260 mg/dl the death rate was 19.9 per 1,000, about two and one half time as high.[26] How this gets reported makes a big difference.

This variation could be expressed by saying that men with higher cholesterols had a death rate 250 percent as high as men with lower cholesterols. Actually the overall increase in death rate was only 1.16 percent spread over a six year period, or about 0.19 percent per year. This is not much of a difference from the effects of what is supposed to be the leading risk factor for heart attacks. And, remember, these results were found in the age group with the most positive association.

This difference certainly is not enough to motivate people to make unpopular and drastic dietary changes for the rest of their lives. There also is no evidence these differences were even related to the blood cholesterol variations. As any first-year biostatistics major learns, associations don't prove cause and effect.

TRYING TO MEASURE POSSIBLE BENEFITS FROM LOWERING BLOOD CHOLESTEROL

Another research group did some calculations based on the assumption that "cholesterol reduction is effective and safe in reducing the risk of death from coronary artery disease." They wrote that for persons aged 20 to 60 who are at low risk, "we calculate a gain in life expectancy of three days to three months from a lifelong program of cholesterol reduction. For persons who are at high risk, the calculated gain ranges from 18 days to 12 months."[27]

The first problem with this study is that the basic assumptions on which it is based were not proven and are now being found to be false. Second, even if efforts to reduce cholesterol levels were safe and effective, the gains are not large enough to motivate people to change their diets radically for the rest of their lives.

ABSENCE OF HEART ATTACKS
IN VERY HIGH RISK MEN

Another exception to the cholesterol theory is seen in people who run very high blood cholesterols because of a dominant hereditary trait. The trait is easy to trace back through a family tree.

The University of Utah School of Medicine screened 1,134 high cholesterol men from 18 families. In four of the families cholesterol levels averaged 352 mg/dl. Men with the abnormal trait averaged having their first heart attack at 42 and dying at 45.[28]

Pedigrees were traced back to four males who were born before 1880 who must have carried the abnormal trait. These men survived to ages 62, 68, 72, and 81. The authors concluded that some unknown healthy lifestyle factors must have protected these men against the expression of the hereditary trait.

It is likely these men were eating the typical high fat diet of Americans of the time. They probably cooked with lard, ate bacon and eggs, other animals, and made sandwiches by spreading bacon grease on their bread.

EXCEPTIONS TO THE CHOLESTEROL THEORY
IN MY PRACTICE

An 86-year-old woman came running into my office one day waving a lab slip in her hand, and I do mean running. She had been in good health all of her life and was still living alone in a self-sufficient manner. Her internist had just presented her with a copy of her blood tests. He had told her she was at a high risk for a heart attack because her blood cholesterol was 360 mg/dl. She caught me in the hall between patients and asked me what she could do to bring her cholesterol level down.

I asked her, "What do you think your cholesterol has been running all of your life?"

She replied, "Well, I suppose it has been about this high for many years, probably most of my life."

I said, "That is a safe assumption. How much damage do you think it has done to you?"

She was forced to answer that no apparent damage had been done. I went on to tell her not to worry about the high cholesterol level and that there were steps she could take to protect herself from a heart attack. However, I assumed it would be hard for her to forget about the test because of all the brainwashing and media hype about cholesterol.

Heart disease dominates the family history of one of my receptionists. Her father had a heart attack and cabbage surgery. Her nephew died of a heart attack at the age of 18 (proven by autopsy). She was aware her own blood cholesterol ran over 300 mg/dl.

In 1990 at age 55 she had a heart scare. She awoke in the middle of the night with crushing chest pain that radiated down her left arm. On her way to the hospital she feared the worst. While an angiogram was being done a surgical team stood by

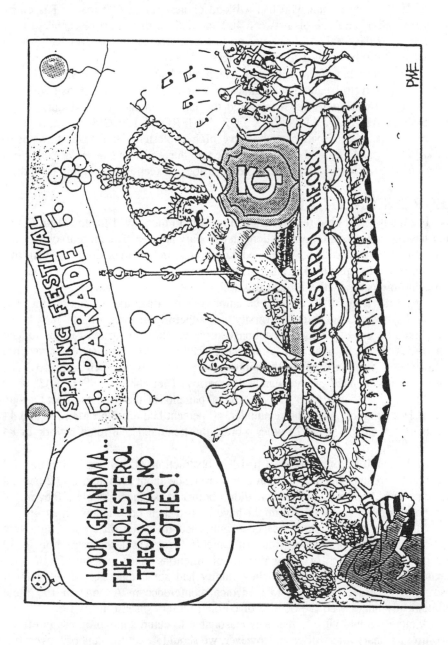

down the hall expecting to do cabbage surgery. To everyone's surprise, the angiogram came out normal showing no obstructions at all. The pain disappeared in a few hours. She went home and has not had a similar episode.

In 1991 I saw a man who had a blood cholesterol of 450 mg/dl. His entire family runs blood cholesterols between 400 and 600, so they must be carriers of the abnormal hereditary trait. Not one person in the entire family has ever had a heart attack, and many have lived to ripe old ages.

On the other end of the scale was a man who had a blood cholesterol of 115. He had suffered a stroke and a heart attack two months before his first visit with me. The low blood cholesterol level triggered the lab's computer to print out, "THIS PATIENT IS AT VERY LOW RISK FOR ATHEROSCLEROSIS."

Every doctor sees patients who have high cholesterol and never have heart attacks. When patients ask about this they are told they must be *one of the exceptions to the cholesterol theory*. There seem to be a lot of exceptions walking around.

REGRESSION STUDIES

For many years lipid researchers had no way to measure if treatment programs were having any effects on obstructions in coronary arteries. The inaccuracies of the angiogram were well known within medicine, so researchers avoided using it for this purpose. When the quantitative angiogram became available in 1977, lipid researchers began to design studies around this test.

The first study that used a variation of the quantitative angiogram was presented by researchers at the University of Southern California. All 162 men in the study had a history of having had cabbage surgery. Blood cholesterol levels ranged from 185 to 350. The treatment group was placed on a low-fat diet plus colestipol (a cholesterol-lowering drug) and niacin (nicotinic acid, a form of vitamin B-3). The control group remained on the Standard American Diet abbreviated (SAD).[29]

At the end of two years, 16 percent of patients in the drug treatment group showed less obstruction. Of the remainder, 40 percent had more obstruction, and 44 percent remained the same. In other words, the treatment plan didn't work in 84 percent of people.

In the control group 2 percent had less obstruction, 60 percent had more, and 38 percent were unchanged. No comments were made about the interesting 2 percent that improved. Apparently researchers didn't bother to ask those people if they might have been doing something that might have helped their obstructions open up.

Another regression study has been published in which different drugs were used.[30] In the most promising group of patients there was less obstruction in 39 percent, and no change or worsening of obstructions in 61 percent. Cholesterol researchers were pleased because they finally had some evidence of reversal of obstructions. These studies led to a medical conference in Arizona in 1992 that optimistically announced the demise of coronary artery disease in its title.

A more rational view is that it is reasonable to claim some progress in efforts to control coronary artery disease. However, we shouldn't get too euphoric over this. One problem with these studies is that they involved the use of drugs that have strong side effects. Many of the drugs are unpleasant to take for long periods of time. Most are expensive in addition to the costs of periodic liver function tests and doctor visits. I, for one, am skeptical about taking a drug for the rest of my life that requires that liver function tests be repeated every six weeks.

Another problem is the overall picture of what happens to people when they take cholesterol-lowering drugs. In the four largest studies published to date heart attack deaths fell by 7 percent. However, deaths from trauma, suicide, and homicides went up by 20 percent. The net change was an *increase* in overall death rates by 7 percent.[31] This is not much to crow about after 40 years of investigations.

LIPID RESEARCHERS WEAR BLINDERS

In late 1991 I had a chance to talk with a lipid (fat) researcher from Stanford University. I asked him about the overall increase in death rates in patients who had been intensively treated with drugs and lower fat diets. He said he was well aware of the problem, but could offer no explanation. I asked him what he thought about the many other exceptions to the cholesterol theory. He looked me squarely in the eye and asked innocently, "What exceptions?"

This shows the degree to which cholesterol researchers have become inbred. There are many promising leads out there that could possibly help solve the heart attack problem, but the lipid people either never hear of them or have no interest in exploring them. They have become experts in the specialized area of fat and cholesterol and communicate only with their own peers. As you will see later they have even developed their own language.

HEART DEATHS WITH LOW CHOLESTEROLS

A consensus conference was held by the National Heart, Lung and Blood Institute of the National Institutes of Health in February, 1992. The meeting was held because a new glitch had surfaced in the cholesterol theory. Large numbers of people were having heart attacks whose blood cholesterols were below 200. In responding to the problem the current director of the Framingham study recommended that physicians should be testing blood HDL (the "good" cholesterol) levels more often, as well as LDL (the "bad" cholesterol) and total cholesterol. If HDL is low, then diet and lifestyle changes can be recommended which may raise it a bit (these efforts are usually not very effective).

Dr. Stephen Hulley of the University of California, San Francisco, stood up and questioned this advice. He said such action would lead to many low risk people being treated with cholesterol-lowering drugs, and this has been shown to *increase* overall death rates by 7 percent.

This debate is reminiscent of what happened at the first consensus conference on cholesterol in 1984. Drs. Peto and Yusuf analyzed 19 diet/drug trials involving 36,000 persons. They concluded that coronary events went down slightly in some studies, but deaths from other causes went up enough to wipe out any gains.[32] It is not logical to continue to ignore findings that are consistently seen, just because they don't fit a pet theory.

Cholesterol is not the only variable that is associated with coronary artery disease. As people become more affluent, heart attack death rates increase. As the number of cars on the street increases, so does heart attack deaths. As the number of fat tummies increases the death rate from heart attacks goes up.

The strongest association ever found has been between the number of television antennas on houses and heart attack death rates. Between 1950 and 1968 the heart attack death rate rose sharply as did the number of television antennas on roof tops. From 1968 to 1990 both the heart attack death rate and number of television antennas came down.

With the beginning of the cable television industry, roof top antennas were no longer needed. If researchers had pursued the association between television antennas and coronary artery disease as vigorously as they did the association between the cholesterol theory and heart attacks, the following may have happened:

A Satirical Look at the Heart Attack and Television Antenna Connection

It came to pass that a new disease fell from the sky and spread throughout the land, the heart attack. The country's best researchers looked at the problem from every angle. Soon an association appeared, backed by the best of circumstantial evidence, something that changed the entire belief system of a generation of physicians. The disease was associated with the number of television antennas on the roofs of homes. As TV antennas increased in number, heart attack deaths increased.

The greatest institutes in the land began scientific studies designed to prove the antenna hypothesis. The theory, stated in simple terms, was this: Putting an antenna on the roof increases risk to the occupant and the higher the antenna the greater the risk. Therefore lowering the level of the antennas (as in cholesterol) was proposed as a logical means of reducing heart attack deaths.

In the first 19 clinical trials researchers lowered antennas on study houses and left them at the same height on control houses. Something *ridiculous* happened in every study. Deaths did not go down. Rather than give up on the theory, researchers became even more relentless. Finally, it was reported in the twentieth trial that for every 1 percent reduction in the height of antennas, heart attack deaths went down by 2 percent. Researchers jumped up and down with joy and proclaimed the theory had at long last been proven.

The National Heart, Lung, Blood, and Antenna Institute of the National Institutes of Health (NHLBAI of NIH) immediately called a consensus meeting. Researchers presented their prize studies for two and a half days. Few were allowed to attend or present papers who were not true believers in the antenna theory.

Some researchers said the diameter of the antenna made a difference. Others speculated parts of the antenna were important, such as the number of prongs. Also studied were thicknesses in wires connecting antennas to the houses as well as grounding. Too many low-density lines (LDL) increased risk, a surplus of high density lines (HDL) decreased risk. Some promoted the hypotheses that there was a difference if the antenna could pick up VHF or UHF. No stone was left unturned.

After two days of conflicting presentations the chairperson took all the bull by the horns and admitted the real consensus had been reached secretly behind closed

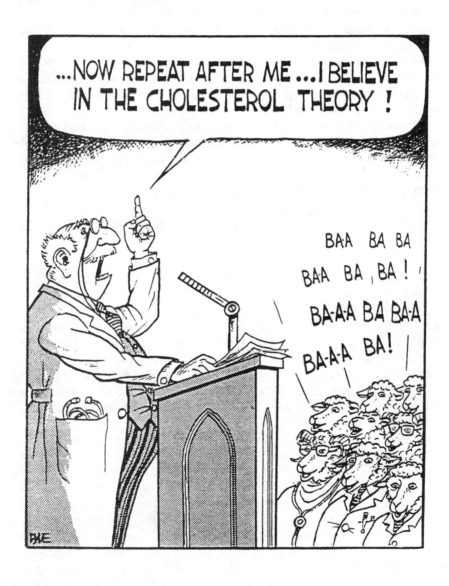

doors two months earlier. The National Antenna Lowering Education Campaign (NALEC) was announced to the press the following morning. The cable TV industry was more than happy to contribute financial support to the campaign.

Over the next few years the rate of deaths from coronary artery disease did go down 7 percent as antennas were lowered. However, the overall death rate went up. Many do-it-yourselfers were falling off of their roof tops trying to remove or lower their dangerous antennas.

This prompted reporters to ask the head of the Porkframe study why attempts to solve the problem seemed only to make things worse. He replied, "What, me worry? Am I supposed to stop treating my patients just because the treatment increases the overall death rate?"

And so it was that more people continued to die of heart attacks than any other cause. Nobody seemed to notice any longer. People slept better at night knowing that a committee of trusted scientists had found a consensus solution for the disease.

OPINIONS OF OTHER EXPERTS ABOUT
THE CHOLESTEROL THEORY

While promoters of the cholesterol theory are strong politically, other independent scientists have raised objections to the lipid (fat) hypothesis. H. Kaunitz, of Columbia University, pointed out that autopsies show that the most severely diseased arteries are found in people who have quite low blood levels of cholesterol.[33]

George V. Mann, of the department of biochemistry, Vanderbilt University, tried to put the last nails in the coffin of the cholesterol theory and bury it in 1977. Mann wrote an article in the *New England Journal of Medicine* titled, "Diet-Heart: End of an Era." He pointed out that the Framingham and Tecumseh studies did not show a cause-effect relationship between cholesterol intake, blood cholesterol levels, and coronary artery disease. He was one of the first to publicize the finding that "risk factors for coronary artery disease don't count after the age of 55." He also warned about dangers from abnormal *trans* fatty acids produced in the processing and hydrogenation of vegetable oils (i.e., margarines.)[34]

In a later article Mann referred to supporters of the cholesterol dogma as the *Heart Mafia* because they received all available research funds aimed at coronary artery disease. He believed the cholesterol theory was a valid hypothesis that was tested and found to be false. Rather than abandon the theory researchers abused the scientific method. He offered a philosophic quotation to explain what developed:

"The moment one has offered an original explanation for a phenomenon which seems satisfactory, that moment affection for his intellectual child springs into existence and, as the explanation grows into a definite theory, his parental affections cluster about his offspring and it grows more and more dear to him...there springs up also unwittingly a pressing of the theory to make it fit the facts and a pressing of the fact to make them fit the theory."[35]

Dr. David Blankenhorn's *regression* study at the University of Southern California begins with the following statement: "The rational for the study was lack of convincing evidence that blood cholesterol lowering has directly beneficial effects on human atherosclerotic lesions (obstructions)." This was written in 1987, three years *after* the consensus conference at NIH declared the cholesterol theory had been proven beyond a reasonable doubt.

Observers from abroad have criticized the cholesterol theory as well. Dr. Martin B. Katan, professor of human nutrition at Wegeningen Agricultural University in the Netherlands, claims the emphasis on the cholesterol blood level in North America has had a major psychological effect. Overnight North Americans awoke and were told 25 percent of them should consider themselves sick with a new disease—*hypercholesterolemia*.

Peter Skrabanek, professor of community health at Trinity College, Dublin, told a recent conference, "Lowering blood cholesterol does not lower overall mortality. None of these studies have shown people live any longer. It is a fascinating sociological phenomenon that some experts, in the face of massive evidence to the contrary, have come up with recommendations based on wishful thinking and dogmatic beliefs. They are guilty of unethical behavior."

William E. Stehbens, professor of pathology at New Zealand's Wellington School of Medicine, claims, "There is no scientific evidence that dietary fat and cholesterol, or even elevated blood cholesterol, causes atherosclerosis. Researchers who fed rats increased amounts of cholesterol did cause fat to accumulate on the walls of their arteries, but these pathological changes are not true atherosclerosis."

Germain J. Brisson, professor of nutrition at Uviversite Laval, Quebec, Canada, was equally blunt in his 1982 book, *Lipids in Human Nutrition*. Brisson stated, "Those who take action and make recommendations as if the lipid hypothesis has been verified are in danger of making a serious mistake. Increasing the consumption of fats rich in polyunsaturated fatty acids and decreasing the intake of cholesterol and fats of animal origin is ineffective in prevention programs designed to reduce the incidence of coronary heart disease."[36]

CONFUSION FROM REDUCTIONISM

You need to be aware of the onslaught of information on the cholesterol theory that is being showered on physicians. In 1991 physicians received a free mail order course (this means drug company sponsored) in recent advances in coronary artery disease.

The course was called, *Arteriosclerosis, a Decade of Progress*. Top names in fat research wrote papers on their various areas of expertise. The vocabulary alone was enough to discourage a non-lipid researcher and keep him or her from wanting to read the course material. It also demonstrated the existing inbreeding among cholesterol/fat experts.

Some of the specialized terms a reader would need to understand to make any sense out of the course material are the following: Apolipoprotein (a), apolipoprotein (b), cholesterol esters, TMA reactive substance, adhesion molecules ELAM, VCAM and ICAM, cytokine activity, tumor necrosis factor, acetyl-LDL or scavenger receptor, arterial tissue macrophage, foam cells, phospholipase A-2, and lipoperoxide radical. You have suffered enough. I refuse to list the other 80 percent.

Of course, any and all of these materials may interact. One paper discussed the functional significance of minimally modified LDL, or MM-LDL. One paragraph went as follows: "Various known adhesion molecules, such as ELAM, VCAM, and ICAM, were suggested as possible candidates for the monocyte-binding substance induced in the endothelium by MM-LDL. ELISA assays performed after treatment of endothelial cells with interleukin-1 (IL-1), a known stimulator of these adhesion molecules, indicated a six to ten fold increase in ELAM on cell surfaces, a five fold increase in VCAM, and a two fold increase in ICAM. MM-LDL, however, failed to induce ELAM or VCAM, and actually depressed ICAM." That may be easy for the researcher to say, but it might as well be ancient Egyptian to most people, including physicians.

In another display of how scientists concentrate on smaller and smaller pieces of a puzzle, cholesterol has been divided into its components, and each of these has been subdivided further. First cholesterol was split into LDL, HDL, and VLDL. Now we are told LDL consists of two parts. There is native LDL, the good guy, and oxidized LDL, the bad guy. HDL has been divided into five numbered parts (I to V) and each of these parts has been subdivided into parts a and b. Now researchers can argue about whether a glass of wine with dinner is good for us because of its effect on HDL-II-b. Aren't you happy you had the opportunity to learn this?

There is an old expression about not being able to tell the forest from the tress. Is it possible that cholesterol researchers have become lost in the trees and can't find their way out?

A TIME BOMB TICKS UNDER THE CHOLESTEROL THEORY

As this manuscript was being prepared additional papers were published that are beginning to dismantle the cholesterol theory. The American Heart Association's own medical journal, *Circulation*, published the largest review of possible risks of blood cholesterol levels on health. The report summarized 19 studies of nearly 650,000 men and women, worldwide.

Cholesterol levels were found to have *no* predictive value in women at any age. Levels of cholesterol between 160 and 240 had no predictive value in men. Men with cholesterols under 160 were 17 percent more likely to die from all causes than men with moderate levels between 160 and 190.[37]

An editorial by Dr. Stephen Hulley, of the University of California, San Francisco, appeared in the same issue. Dr. Hulley stated that routine screening for blood cholesterols had no value in women or children. About the only time screening might be of value was in men who had already had a heart attack or were at high risk of developing coronary artery disease.[38] Actually, this can't really be called *screening*. These men would have these tests done routinely because of current or possible future problems. Hence, the massive cholesterol screening program is of no value.

Researchers have reacted to the report in various ways. Some have automatically defended the screening program. Others have called for an elimination of

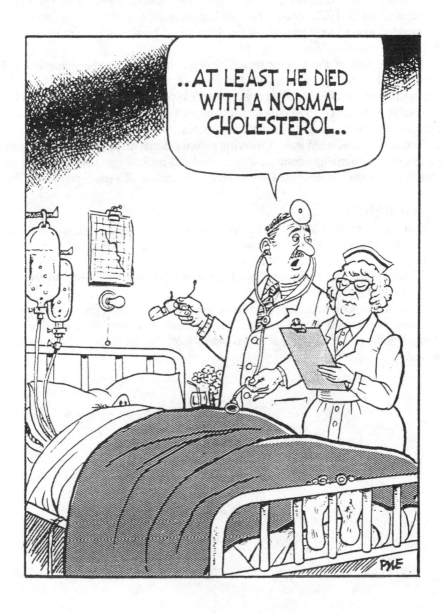

routine screening and treatment of people with high levels of cholesterol. Such an action would have major effects on the $20 billion-plus a year industry that has grown up around cholesterol screening tests and cholesterol-lowering drugs.

Another article detrimental to the cholesterol theory appeared in the *British Medical Journal* in 1992. Twenty-two studies were evaluated in which efforts had been made to lower blood cholesterol levels to see if heart attack death rates would fall.

In about half of the articles reviewed death rates fell, in the remainder they increased. Statistical errors were found in most of the articles that were claimed to be supportive of the cholesterol theory. The article pointed out there is so much bias in this subject that since 1970 only articles supportive of the cholesterol theory have been cited as references in other medical articles.

The author concluded that, "Lowering serum (blood) cholesterol concentrations does not reduce mortality (death) and is unlikely to prevent coronary heart disease. Claims of the opposite are based on preferential citation of supportive trials."[39]

CONCLUSION

You don't have to look very far to find exceptions to the cholesterol theory. Early animal studies that launched the theory were flawed. Reports of later studies in humans have been slanted. Statistics have been misinterpreted to support the theory since 1970. The theory developed a life of its own and has risen to the level of a religious dogma.

It is time to look into other promising areas that have been ignored because of preexisting biases and tunnel vision. The cholesterol theory is a fraud on the American public. At long last it is beginning to look like the theory will be exposed as a scam.

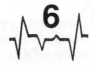

6

WINNERS AND LOSERS FROM THE CHOLESTEROL THEORY

We are all born brave, trusting and greedy, and most of us remain greedy.

Mignon McLaughlin

Controversies produce winners and losers. Organizations and commercial interests benefiting from the cholesterol theory include processors of vegetable oils and margarines, the drug industry, the medical industry, the American Heart Association, and the National Heart, Lung and Blood Institute of the National Institutes of Health. Losers include the producers of eggs, beef, dairy products and the public.

IMPACT ON THE AMERICAN HEART ASSOCIATION AND THE NATIONAL INSTITUTES OF HEALTH

The American Heart Association and the cholesterol theory needed each other. The American Heart Association is the major fund-raising organization for heart disease research in the United States. In trying to reduce the impact of the number one killer disease in the Western world, the American Heart Association assumed a large responsibility. With this responsibility came a pressing need to find solutions to the problem. However, the American Heart Association is dependent on donations from the public for its very existence, and this can lead to problems.

It is difficult to be the self proclaimed expert organization in the field of heart disease, then one dismal year after another have no progress to report. This makes fund-raising difficult. Imagine how you would respond to someone knocking on your door with the following pitch: "I am collecting money for the American Heart Association. We have been working on the heart attack problem for many years. We haven't found a dam thing yet, but give us more money anyway." It is easier to raise funds by claiming progress and success, though the progress may be nothing more than pie in the sky.

For many years doctors didn't claim to have any plausible explanation for why people had heart attacks. The problem was viewed as if heart attacks fell from the sky onto normal people for no reason. When the American Heart Association

77

accepted the cholesterol theory, fund-raisers at long last had the opportunity to claim progress in fighting the disease. The next step was to educate the public about alleged benefits of a low fat/low cholesterol diet.

Although a branch of the Federal Government, the National Heart, Lung and Blood Institute of the National Institutes of Health found itself in much the same position. Its task has been to oversee and fund research in coronary artery disease. In so doing it has played a strong role in the direction any research would take. Its directors must have been ecstatic when scientists reported they had found an association between cholesterol and coronary artery disease. Tunnel vision and biases took over from there.

IMPACT ON THE FOOD INDUSTRY

The cholesterol theory has had a dramatic impact on certain segments of the food industry. Some producers found they could use the cholesterol theory to their financial advantage. Others were hit in the pocketbook for no good reason.

Oils and Margarines

Animal products are the only sources of saturated fats and cholesterol in the diet. Cholesterol is not found in vegetables, seeds, and grains. You would have no idea this was the case from the advertising of vegetable oils and margarines.

In their advertisements margarine and vegetable oil companies focus attention on this absence of cholesterol in their products. The implication is made that eating their products will be good for your heart because they contain no cholesterol. Each brand of vegetable oil proudly proclaims its product contains no cholesterol, as if to imply that competing brands do. This is nothing more than a form of deception in advertising.

The current advertising trend is getting even more ridiculous. Some breads are being advertised as containing no cholesterol. Soon we may see products such as motor oil and hair spray being advertised as containing no cholesterol. Such claims would be about as useful.

When human feeding studies showed a low fat diet plus the use of a certain vegetable oil reduced blood cholesterol levels by a certain percentage, manufacturers exploited the finding. Other studies have been ignored that showed cancer rates went up when animals ate less saturated fats and more polyunsaturated oils. Also ignored was an interesting human study. As consumption of corn oil was increased, blood cholesterol levels fell, but he heart attack death rate increased.

Beef

The beef industry suffered in the early days of the cholesterol theory. Both sales prices and volumes of sales fell. However, because Americans have a strong affection for beef, sales volumes slowly recovered back to about where they were.

The industry has condescended to the political clout of the cholesterol theory. In 1991 the beef industry ran an advertising campaign based on the fat content of a three ounce serving of beef. This step looked ridiculous. Most Americans would consider themselves to be wimps if they served themselves such a small fragment.

Real men would never put up with such a dinky tidbit.

The Egg, Public Enemy Number One

The egg industry took the cholesterol theory on the chin. Per capita consumption of eggs has fallen by 40 percent since 1950 and remains depressed. Many Americans regard eating eggs as being worse than flunking a blood test for AIDS or drinking hemlock.

No research has ever shown fresh eggs are harmful to humans when they are cooked as they would be for a typical breakfast. In one study when human volunteers ate as many as 35 eggs per week, blood cholesterol levels remained constant.

Several years ago nutritionists developed a quality ranking system for foods according to overall nutritional value. They gave the egg a perfect rating of 100. After giving eggs the highest rating, they proceeded to tell us not to eat them because of their high cholesterol content!

In the 1960 the egg industry tried to fight the cholesterol theory with a frontal attack by forming the National Commission on Egg Nutrition. The organization ran advertisements stating there was no scientific evidence that eating eggs had been shown to increase the risk of heart attacks. The statement was perfectly true, but that small detail didn't matter.

The president of the American Heart Association complained about the ads to the Federal Trade Commission, requesting that they be banned. The Federal Trade Commission brought charges against the National Committee on Egg Nutrition claiming they had used unfair and deceptive practices.

A trial was held. Similar to a lynching, the Federal Trade Commission presided as accuser, judge, and jury. The FTC ruled that the National Committee on Egg Nutrition had made false and misleading statements. The judge believed the testimony of scientists who were totally committed to the cholesterol theory.[1] As a result the egg became a convicted felon, an official enemy of the public. It took a bum rap.

The Dairy Industry

The dairy industry has experienced two serious threats to its economic stability since World War II. First came a health scare related to the radioactive compound, strontium 90. Researchers needed to select an animal to measure how much radioactivity was entering the food supply from atmospheric testing of atomic weapons over the Pacific Ocean in the early 1950s. Any domestic animal could have been chosen because the results would have been the same. The radioactive compound would have been found in human milk as well. Unfortunately for the dairy industry, the cow got the nod.

When the public heard that researchers had found strontium 90 in cow's milk, dairy sales fell and stayed low for several years. As the memory of that scare was beginning to fade away and sales were beginning to recover, along came the second part of the double whammy, the cholesterol scare. Sales fell off again.

The dairy industry was quick on its feet. The problem was solved by separating milk into different portions and selling them separately. New low fat products were created such as skimmed milk and 2 percent low fat milk.

IMPACT ON THE DRUG INDUSTRY

The drug industry was more than happy to support the cholesterol theory. One of the assumptions of the theory is that reductions in serum cholesterol, achieved by any means, will end up being beneficial. Various companies began to develop a series of products that lower blood cholesterol levels through one mechanism or another.

The first cholesterol-lowering drug on the market was MER-29. First released in the early 1960s, MER-29 didn't stay on the market long. The drug caused a high rate of cataract formation which led to its withdrawal from the market after a couple of years. As frequently occurs with drugs, serious side effects did not come to the attention of the FDA until the product had been on the market for a year or two.

Other cholesterol-lowering drugs soon followed. Now there are several categories of cholesterol-lowering agents from which to choose. Most still have troublesome side effects, usually interference with normal liver function or cataract formation.

Another problem with cholesterol-lowering drugs is their cost. Total cost for a cholesterol-lowering medication, laboratory testing, and doctor visits can easily run as high as $3,000 during the first year, then $2,000 per year, forever. Merck reports wholesale sales of lovastatin are currently running over $1 billion per year and soon are expected to double.

Therefore, drug companies with cholesterol-lowering products on the market, or in research stages, have a lot to gain from the cholesterol theory. Ignored by physicians and the FDA are four large studies that have shown overall death rates actually go *up* when people take cholesterol-lowering drugs (see Chapter 5).

IMPACT ON THE MEDICAL INDUSTRY

Doctors accepted the cholesterol theory with reluctance. One reason for this delay was a long held general belief among physicians that we can pour any type of junk food down our gullets and it will have no effect on our health.

Two events changed this attitude. The public took more of an interest in the cholesterol issue, and doctors found out that treating elevated blood cholesterol was good for their incomes. With the beginning of the National Cholesterol Education Program in 1985, more and more physicians decided to become crusaders in the war against cholesterol.

As a result of the National Cholesterol Education program, cholesterol screening became available in shopping malls and other convenient public settings. When high blood cholesterol levels are found, people are referred to their personal physicians. If repeat tests confirm a high cholesterol level, treatment to lower the cholesterol level is advised.

The first level of treatment for an elevated blood cholesterol is to put patients on the American Heart Association's diet. After that fails the doctor is advised to pull out the prescription pad and place the patient on one of the cholesterol-lowering drugs. With follow up visits and monthly laboratory tests, billings increase.

The physician is also rewarded emotionally for following this protocol. The doctor receives strokes from experts who keep repeating over and over that this represents state of the art, high-quality, preventive medicine. It is no wonder the medical profession cooperates.

It is probable most doctors have never read the medical literature on which the cholesterol theory is based. Usually, they are too busy to look into controversial issues personally. They tend to follow the policies of organizations in which they have placed their trust, such as the American Heart Association and drug companies.

CONCLUSIONS

A coalition of vested interests supports the cholesterol theory. Supporters include the American Heart Association, the National Heart, Lung and Blood Institute of the National Institutes of Health, drug companies who manufacture cholesterol-lowering drugs, the producers of vegetable oils and margarines, and the medical industry. This is a powerful alliance. It will be most difficult to remove ourselves from the influence of the cholesterol theory simply because the facts show it is false.

7

**METHODS THAT
REALLY HELP**

*Men occasionally stumble over the truth, but most pick themselves
up and hurry off as if nothing had happened.*

Winston Churchill

In previous chapters we discussed cholesterol related therapies, angioplasties, bypasses and balloon procedures. Although these procedures and concepts are in common usage, a review of the medical literature shows they are seldom indicated and have had no impact on reducing death rates from coronary artery disease. Other more promising concepts and approaches exist, but have remained virtually unknown.

In this chapter we will examine lifestyle and health practices of groups of people who have remained free of coronary artery disease. We also will look at several programs that have really helped patients with coronary artery disease, including the first and only one proven to reverse arterial obstructions in a high percentage of people.

STUDIES AMONG PRIMITIVE LIFESTYLE PEOPLE

As a general pattern, primitive lifestyle people remained free of our modern diseases of physical degeneration until they had contact with the outside world. They drank polluted water and had poor hygiene. As a result they had high infant death rates and suffered from many preventable infectious diseases.

In contrast, they did not experience diseases of physical degeneration such as heart attacks, high blood pressure, strokes, diabetes, tooth decay, acne, osteoporosis and a long list of other conditions that fill modern hospitals. Europeans have referred to these conditions as *diseases of civilization*, because, with rare exceptions, they were not seen in primitive lifestyle people regardless how old they lived.

Some people have tried to say these diseases were not seen because primitive people didn't live long enough to develop them. They support this by pointing out that the *average* life expectancy in these areas was often only 35 to 40. This is really nothing more than a misinterpretation of statistics. The *average* life expectancy was pulled down because about 40 percent of babies born alive were dying of infections related to dirty water and poor hygiene before their second birthday. The remainder of the people died between the ages of 50 and 90. Almost nobody died between the ages of two and fifty except for cases of burns and trauma (or during yellow fever epidemics).

In any event, the health of primitive lifestyle people fell apart after outsiders arrived on the scene. Many people have described this decline in health, but *very* few figured out the reasons for this drastic shift in the disease pattern. Unlocking the mechanism of this disease pattern shift has great implications for the future health of mankind.

I have observed that this pattern of illness among primitive lifestyle people does not impress physicians unless they have seen it first hand, and *also* have had some awareness of what was going on. Many have traveled to or worked in areas of the world that have had this pattern, but few doctors have appreciated what they have seen.

I consider myself fortunate to have had two encounters with this pattern. For one year, starting in 1965, I treated Indians in a government hospital high in the Andes mountains of Ecuador. Modern degenerative diseases were almost absent in the Indian population. The other exposure to this pattern of disease was in Hainan Province, China, and is described below.

SURVEYS OF PRIMITIVE LIFESTYLE PEOPLE

In preparation for the opening of a medical school in East Africa in 1930, British doctors surveyed the disease pattern of random samples of 3,000,000 Bantu natives. The professors wanted to aim the teaching curriculum at prevalent diseases of the area. Physical examinations were performed, as well as EKGs, blood pressure measurements, and urine and blood tests for sugar.

Not one Bantu was found to have any evidence of diabetes, high blood pressure, stroke, or coronary artery disease. During this time physicians performed autopsies on many Bantus and found no evidence of heart attacks.

Thirty years later all of these conditions were beginning to appear. These findings were described by Hugh C. Trowell, a British physician who practiced among the Bantus from 1930 to 1960. The disease pattern shift occurred during his tenure in Africa and he was astute enough to connect changes in diseases with changes in the diet.[1]

THE DENTAL CONNECTION

Weston Price, D.D.S. was one of the first people to blame the development of diseases of physical degeneration on the entry of modern refined foods into the diet. Price was a retired dentist who wanted to devote the remainder of his life to studying why people developed tooth decay. In a radical departure from the norm, Price decided to study people who did not have decay to see what they might be doing that made them different.

Between 1930 and 1940 Price traveled over 60,000 miles examining the dental status of natives in many areas of the world.[2] He found that the more difficulty he had reaching an isolated native population, the less those people suffered from tooth decay and other diseases of civilization.

Totally isolated natives had almost no tooth decay. Typically all 32 teeth came in straight. He had to examine four adults to find one decayed tooth. People were robust into old age with good eyesight, strong physiques, sharp minds, and they did not lose their teeth.

When Price could reach an area easily by truck, bus, or trading ship, he found a different pattern. If contact with the outside world had been recent, he found dramatic changes in children. Children under a certain age had more narrow jaws than either parent, and decay rates ran between 30 to 50 percent of all teeth. Children over that age had perfect jaw structure and almost no tooth decay.

The age break corresponded to how many years the store had been open. After developing this finding, Price was able to astound the native chiefs of new areas he visited. He would first examine the mouths of children and recorded their ages, then accurately tell the chief the year their store had opened.

Price reported a sad finding. After the entry of what he called the *foods of modern commerce*, a new problem began to be seen. Some people developed oral infections and in the absence of treatment many developed into abscesses. As dentists were not available to drain these abscesses, people began to resort to suicide as a means of ending their perpetual pain. A high price was paid for the pleasure of eating what we call *junk food*.

Price identified the culprits in the diet as refined carbohydrates (i.e., sugar, white flour, white rice) found in such items as soda pop, jams, marmalade, white flour crackers and candy bars. If a mother began to consume these products during a pregnancy, her next baby and subsequent children would grow up with a high decay rate and crooked teeth. All previous children from the same marriage had normal jaw structure and teeth. If a woman later rejected modern refined foods, subsequent children were once again normal.

The frightening finding was that only a small percentage of the diet had to shift to refined foods to trigger these changes. In most cases the majority of food consumed continued to be the same as had always been grown and gathered in the area. The amount of store food purchased was limited by pitifully low wages.

Price's book contains pages and pages of photographs of natives showing their good or bad teeth. Also included are photographs of 500-year-old skulls of Inca Indians from Peru. None of the skulls showed any evidence of decay or crooked teeth.

Every time I see teenagers with crooked teeth or braces I am reminded of Dr. Price and the sad thought that crooked teeth are preventable. In this modern world we almost expect children to have crooked teeth and to need orthodontia services. In the past there was little need for that dental specialty. If an orthodontist had set up a practice among primitive lifestyle people, he would have starved.

THE EPIDEMIOLOGY OF CLEAVE

The next pioneer to make a strong contribution to our knowledge was British epidemiologist, T.L. Cleave, M.D. I believe Cleave deserves the credit for solving the riddle of the onset of degenerative diseases more than anybody else. Cleave worked at the Naval Medical School in London, England. In the 1940s he published a series of papers about his discoveries and finally wrote a book summarizing his findings.[3]

Cleave found that the entry of refined carbohydrates into the diets of primitive lifestyle people led to the onset of diseases of physical degeneration (including heart attacks). The tricky part was that the effect was delayed. He found the disease pattern shift occurred about 20 to 30 years after modern foods began to be consumed, a delay he called an *incubation period*. This delay made the entire concept abstract. The delay also made the idea impossible to prove in human experiments because you can't lock humans up for a lifetime and conduct studies. The concept has been reproduced in animal feeding experiments. It is also consistent with knowledge gained in biochemistry, inborn errors of metabolism, and certain genetic disorders.

In hundreds of locations around the world from which information was available, Cleave never found a single exception to this pattern. This may be the most consistent finding in the entire field of medicine.

NORTHERN YUKON TERRITORY ESKIMOS

Eskimos of the Northern Yukon Territory of Canada were nomadic food gathers until 1955. In that year the Defense Early Warning (DEW) system was built to try to detect Russian missiles coming over the North Pole. Eskimos from all across northern Canada and Alaska took jobs building air fields and radar stations.

The Eskimos gave up their food gathering ways and moved to town. Overnight they made a switch from a diet of 100 percent natural fresh foods to 100 percent modern store foods which were shipped in from outside. Instead of the usual incubation period of 30 years, the disease pattern shift described by Cleave was condensed to only 10 to 15 years.

Women began to suffer gallbladder attacks and develop diabetes. Men developed coronary artery disease. Children developed tooth decay and acne. None of these conditions had been seen in these people before.

A team of doctors from Edmonton, Alberta, described these changes. The doctors had been providing medical care in a regional hospital in the area for many years. These disease pattern changes occurred right under their noses. Almost as they watched. They were so impressed they wrote an article about their observations titled, *When the Eskimo Comes to Town*, which was published in a major nutrition journal.[4]

WORLD WAR II

War conditions forced a severe change in diet patterns in England during World War II. Even though conditions were severe, specific health improvements were seen. During a four year period in the middle of the war, death rates for both heart attacks and diabetes fell by 50 percent.

As usual, when something good happens, supporters of various concepts swoop down like vultures to take the credit. Believers in the cholesterol theory have claimed that the drop in heart attack deaths must have occurred because consumption of animal products went down during the war. However, many other drastic shifts in the food supply were occurring that the cholesterol supporters conveniently overlook.

Sugar was rationed and consumption fell drastically because of shipping hazards on the high seas. The British Government made a decision to conserve energy by not sifting whole wheat flour into white flour. This forced people to eat more nourishing whole wheat products. The government encouraged people to plant victory gardens and the intake of fresh vegetables increased. In many ways the diet reverted to the way it had been in the past before the advent of refined foods.[5]

THE PRITIKIN PROGRAM

Nathan Pritikin was an engineer by trade. When he failed a treadmill test in 1958, he asked his doctor what he could do to reverse his heart condition. Angiograms, cabbages and balloon jobs were not yet available, or he might have been talked into one of more of those procedures. As usual the doctor had nothing to offer. Pritikin was told to come back when he had more trouble.

Pritikin researched the medical literature on coronary artery disease and learned about the absence of the disease in primitive lifestyle people. He found that most primitive lifestyle people of the world at fresh foods and very few animal products (he never mentioned successful cultures that ate high fat diets).

Pritikin concluded that the Heart Association recommendation of reducing fat intake from 40 to 30 percent of the diet was not going to be a big enough change to improve anything. Because of the popularity of the cholesterol theory, he put himself on a vegetarian diet containing only 10 percent fat. His condition gradually improved.

In the mid-1970s the *Pritikin Longevity Center* was opened in Santa Barbara, California. Under medical supervision, patients entered a four week program. This involved an extremely low fat diet, the elimination of processed foods, and walking up to six miles a day at a leisurely pace.

Favorable things began to happen to people in the program. Angina pains usually went away. People who were too ill to walk when they arrived soon found they could begin to ambulate. Overweight people lost weight. EKGs and treadmill tests frequently improved. Many people began to enjoy living again. The live-in program currently is offered in Santa Monica, California.

Pritikin was a fanatic about keeping fat out of the diet. He claimed there was enough fat in lettuce and other vegetables to suffice. Colleagues of mine have described seeing compulsive Pritikin Program patients become deficient in essential fatty acids after they have been on the diet about two years. These people entered the office looking gaunt, with skin that was dry, droopy, pale, gray, and flaky. Fortunately this complication was seldom seen because most people find it difficult to keep fat intake down to the 10 percent level without cheating.

I remember how physician friends of mine criticized the program when we first heard about it. The usual comment was that improvements described in heart patients were impossible. Doctors as a group are a negative, fatalistic bunch. Most believed improvements in cardiac status could not be achieved by any means, let alone through something as simple as a change in diet and walking.

The biggest objection the medical establishment has voiced about the Pritikin Program is the lack of convincing evidence showing obstructions in arteries have opened up. Improvements frequently are seen in walking distances, anginal attacks, EKGs, and the insulin requirements of diabetics. Unfortunately, Pritikin Program patients have never been evaluated with the quantitative angiogram. This is a problem with modern medicine. Obvious signs of improvement don't count unless the right test has documented changes on a piece of paper.

Pritikin had the last laugh. He died in 1985 at the age of 69. He lived with a malignant lymphoma during his last 27 years. At autopsy his coronary arteries were described as resembling a newborn baby's. This was remarkable for a man his age who had a history of documented coronary artery disease with or without a malignancy.[6]

While Pritikin was alive physicians laughed at his efforts. Pritikin had the wrong diploma on the wall. He was an engineer, not a member of the medical fraternity. His program has become easier for doctors to accept after his death. Some cardiologists now hire nutritional counselors to work in their offices instructing patients in the Pritikin Program.

REVERSING HEART DISEASE A LA ORNISH

Dean Ornish, M.D., is affiliated with the University of California Medical School in San Francisco. Over several years Ornish completed preliminary studies to see if diet and lifestyle changes could alter the course of coronary artery disease. He found heart patients' conditions could be improved, but needed a way to prove his findings.

Ornish reported results of what he called *The Lifestyle Heart Trial* in 1990 in both the medical journal *Lancet* and a large book.[7, 8] The CBS-TV program, *60 Minutes*, and an hour long episode of the NOVA series on Public Television presented his program to the public.

Patients with significant coronary artery disease problems were randomly divided into two groups. The lifestyle change group followed a vegetarian diet that contained only 10 percent fat. People in that group also stopped smoking, meditated one hour per day (after receiving expert instruction), exercised, and underwent lengthy group therapy sessions.

The control group followed the standard American Heart Association diet (fat intake under 30 percent of diet and cholesterol less than 300 mg per day) and received routine medical care from their own physicians. All patients received a quantitative angiogram at the beginning of the program and after one year.

Patients on Ornish's program did far better in relieving symptoms and opening their obstructions than control patients. Most study patients were free of angina within one month of starting the program. Those who complied with the demands of the program improved more than patients who were not so strict.

In patients with the worst obstructions, the diameter of partially blocked arteries increased (improved) an average of 8.6 percent. That is almost enough to double the surface area of the opening of an artery and improve blood flow tremendously.

In patients in the control group who had the most severe blockages, the diameter of partially blocked arteries narrowed (worsened) by an average of 4.4 percent. problems with angina pain also increased during the year, and medication use increased. This should not have been surprising because no previous studies have shown the diet of the American Heart Association works.

One man in the lifestyle group died during the 12 months of study. He elected not to participate in group therapy sessions and did not practice meditation. Instead of attending those sessions he chose to go to the gym to pursue a program of vigorous exercise. About nine months into the program he died suddenly while working out on a rowing machine. After this unfortunate death his wife found an application form in the glove box of his car. He was planning to complete in a 10K running competition.

Though this study produced the best, documented results to date, physician response has been mixed. Nobody has doubted that obstructions did in fact open up. Some experts complimented Ornish on his work, then stated their opinion that most Americans would never follow such a time consuming regime that changes almost everything in their lives. This attitude of doctors automatically precludes them from presenting a program such as this to their patients.

In many people's minds this omission amounts to malpractice because of a failure to provide a patient with enough information to give an *informed consent* for a surgical procedure. At least one lawsuit in California occurred over this failure to fully inform a patient of options before a cabbage surgery was done.

Ornish agrees the program will not appeal to everyone. Most Americans want a quick fix in the form of a pill or surgery. But he feels more patients should be informed of this option.

Other experts have been more critical, pointing out that Ornish can't tell which part of the program produced the results. Those critics are following the classical thinking in medicine that a single *magic bullet* treatment must exist for each individual disease.

What Ornish's program proves is that the body has the ability to heal itself and reverse coronary artery disease. Our bodies have an amazing ability to heal if only we could stop doing things that get in the way. After publication of Ornish's paper and book, patients continue to come to my office and say their doctors have told them coronary artery disease can't be reversed. Ornish's work proves they are wrong.

A COMPARISON OF ORNISH'S PROGRAM
AND REGRESSION STUDIES

Experts in coronary artery disease are now referring to three programs that have demonstrated it is possible for obstructions to reverse themselves and open up. In the first study a cholesterol-lowering drug was used and 16 percent of patients were shown to have less obstruction.[9] In the second study a cholesterol-lowering drug and niacin (a form of vitamin B-3) were used and 39 percent of patients had less obstruction.[10] The third is Ornish's study described above.

When these reports are compared, the best results by far were seen in the Ornish study. Ornish's program worked in 85 percent of patients compared to only 39 percent in the best of the other two studies. In patients with blockages of 50 percent or greater, arteries opened 8.6 percent in one year in the Ornish study compared to 6.4 percent in two and one half years in the second best study. Also, in the Ornish study, patients were not required to put up with the side effects and risks of the drugs used in the other studies.

HAINAN ISLAND, CHINA

China is a large country with a diversity of climates and dietary practices. Disease patterns also vary widely. The death rate from coronary artery disease is low in China (50 per 100,000 population) compared to more developed countries. Almost all deaths from heart attacks occur in urban areas. In cities, coronary artery disease is second only to cancer as a leading cause of death.

Western trained doctors in China give lip service to the cholesterol theory because they read about it in medical journals from the West. However, total fat intake is only 20 percent in the cities and 10 percent in the countryside. Because the overall death rate is low, doctors don't view the problem as very serious and everyone continues to eat what he or she likes.[11]

Hainan province is a very special situation, worthy of some intensive study by international medical organizations. For many years Hainan Island was an ignored part of Canton Province. While the area around Canton (Guangzhao) developed economically, Hainan Island was left in its pristine state. To help speed development, the central government made Hainan a separate province in 1987.

Now, 8,000,000 people live on Hainan Island. The climate is tropical, similar to Hong Kong (300 miles to the east). Over 90 percent of people live on farms. Health statistics from 1990 reveal some unusual patterns.

Average life expectancy at birth is 87, a full ten years longer than anywhere else in the world. Pregnancy related problems don't occur. The infant death rate is 13 per 1,000 live births, compared to 9 per 1,000 live births in the United States (the infant death rate refers to how many babies born alive die from all causes in their first year, per 1,000 live births).

Absent are birth defects, premature births, or significant problems with new-born infants. Therefore there is no need for neonatologists or intensive care nurseries. Non-tropical infectious diseases fill the list of the top ten causes of death. Coronary artery disease is rare.

These observations show Hainan has defied the worldwide disease pattern shift described by Cleave. Throughout history the health of primitive lifestyle people disintegrated about 20 to 30 years after contact with the outside world. The common observation is that infectious diseases, related to a lack of clean water and personal hygiene, almost vanish, only to be replaced by chronic degenerative diseases in about 20-plus years.

I have visited the farming people of Hainan on several occasions. Their living conditions make cleanliness difficult. Pigs and chickens walk in and out of homes of poor people, and human waste is used as fertilizer. However, people are clean when it counts. They may lack modern indoor plumbing, but custom dictates that hands be washed before eating.

Hainan people stem or stir fry food in super-heated woks. Everything is cooked except fruit which is peeled immediately before eating. As a general rule, nothing is overcooked.

The Chinese developed a practice 2,000 years ago of not drinking water unless it has first been boiled. The practice remains useful because potable water systems existent only in newer hotels. When my Chinese host visited my home in 1987, he refused to drink our pure well water, fresh from the tap. On later visits he learned he could trust the water.

The people of Hainan put a high priority on the freshness of food. If you want a chicken dinner, the first step is to catch and kill a chicken. In the fish market people select fish that are swimming around in tanks, then take them home swimming in buckets of water. When I told Hainan people many of the fish Americans eat have been frozen, their mouths fell open in disbelief. One of them questioned, "You would eat a fish that has been frozen?"

Farmers pick vegetables in the morning and sell them from small carts in farmers' markets a few hours later. Supermarkets don't exist. They only foods sold in containers are sauces for seasoning which are available in glass bottles. Rice is polished much less than in the United States. This causes the part consumed by humans to contain more nutrients than white rice in the United States. These patterns make the food safe to eat, yet preserve close to 100 percent of the nutritional value of the fresh product.

Other factors may play a role in this unusual pattern of health. Farmers don't use synthetic fertilizers, herbicides, or pesticide sprays, mostly because of their high costs. Vegetables remain lush and healthy. Top soils continue to increase in depth and quality as farmers recycle all waste products. This is a sharp contrast with the problem of the loss of top soils in the United States due to mono-culture and chemical farming practices.

Whatever the people of Hainan are doing is working for them. They may now have the best overall health pattern of any people in the world. They should be studied thoroughly before progress arrives and changes everything. The diet is already beginning to change now with the entry of high sugar content soft drinks and candy.

EDTA CHELATION THERAPY

Dr. G. was only 30 when he began to suffer from angina. Over the next three years symptoms got so bad he had to close his medical office. At the time Dr. G. was a believer in the powers of modern medicine with its wonder drugs and surgical advances. Therefore, it was logical for G. to go directly to the *ivory tower*. He made an appointment to see top heart specialists at a nearby university medical center.

After performing tests available in 1968, experts told Dr. G. he had severe coronary artery disease, a diagnosis it didn't take a rocket scientist to deduce. They advised nitroglycerin tablets as needed for anginal pains, and a lot of rest. The advice was of little value because Dr. G. was already doing these things and the problem was getting worse. He asked if modern medicine had anything more to offer.

Cabbage surgery was in its developmental stages. The experts told Dr. G. he could have the experimental surgical procedure to *revascularize* his heart. The use of that buzz word has always added a feeling of optimism to the procedure. Dr. G. was not fooled. He asked what the operative death rate was running. The experts told him it was 50 percent. Dr. G. walked out of the medical center and was never seen there again.

Dr. G. was an avid reader with a photographic memory. He buried himself in the medical library, reading everything he could find about coronary artery disease. He stumbled into articles describing treatments with a metal binding compound, ethylene-diamine-tetra-acetic acid, or EDTA for short.

EDTA

EDTA was being used as a treatment for lead poisoning and had become the treatment of choice for that condition. In the early 1950s some people being treated for lead poisoning told their doctors that their anginal pains were improving as they received more treatments. This led to about ten years of research on the relationship between EDTA and arterial disease. Scores of papers were published, all favorable. In the early 1960s the product insert for EDTA from Abbott Laboratories listed arteriosclerosis as an indication for its use.

Then three things happened to drastically change the situation. First, the scientist who was the leading proponent of the treatment was killed in an auto accident. Second, Abbott's patent was running out. Third, the FDA put into effect new requirements of proof of efficacy for drugs.

Abbott Laboratories had no choice but to drop arteriosclerosis as an indication in the product insert. No drug company is going to spend millions of dollars researching a generic drug it can't profit from and control.

For mysterious and apparently political reasons the treatment fell into disfavor. All articles published up to that time, with the exception of one, described improvements in a high percentage of patients. That exception makes interesting reading.

The body of the article describes how patients were improving from chelation therapy. Even the next to last paragraph states chelation is an excellent treatment for small artery disease. This is followed by a summary paragraph stating the treatment is no good.[12]

Arline Brecher reported in her book *Forty Something Forever*, that the insurance industry bribed the authors to produce a negative report of the study. This was done to protect insurance companies from losing money from the procedure. Insurance companies could go bankrupt if they were hit broadside in the middle of a policy year by millions of dollars of bills for a new procedure.[13]

After treatment methods are attacked by establishment medicine, they die quickly. By 1968 only two doctors in the United States were openly using chelation therapy in their practices. Dr. G. visited one of them in Alabama and learned how to treat himself. He gave himself more than 20 intravenous infusions of EDTA, along with magnesium and other nutrients. He also placed himself on a high complex carbohydrate diet, fresh foods, vitamins and minerals, and an exercise program. All junk foods were eliminated.

His angina gradually disappeared completely. Now, 25 years later, he has no symptoms of coronary artery disease. Dr. G. is a hyperactive sort of person, works hard, plays hard, and is on the go 18 hours a day. When the band begins to play fast music at a dance he grabs his partner and heads for the dance floor.

Over 1,000 doctors in the United States currently offer chelation therapy in their practices. Twice a year the American College of Advancement of Medicine (ACAM) sponsors training programs in chelation therapy for physicians. Interest is so high that demand for this instruction currently exceeds capacity. The medical establishment has installed a permanent black cloud over the therapy and considers it to be nothing more than a form of quackery.

Opponents claim chelation therapy for circulation disorders is ineffective, expensive, risky, and can cause death. They don't accept the favorable results reported in older studies on the grounds that the studies do not meet current research standards. Opponents claim that no recent studies supporting chelation therapy can be found in peer reviewed medical journals. Therefore, they consider chelation to be experimental and view offering it to the public to be unethical.

Proponents say one recent double-blind study from Brazil has shown chelation does work.[14] Everyone agrees more such studies are needed. However, many significant favorable clinical studies exist that were not double-blinded. Major journals have not accepted these articles because of biases of physicians on their editorial boards. Therefore, the articles have appeared in journals such as the *American Journal of Holistic Medicine*, and ACAM's own journal, *the Journal of Advancement in Medicine*. These journals are not cross-indexed into medical computer banks.

CHELATION STUDIES

An isotope study reported in 1989 showed improved blood flow to the brain in 80 to 85 percent of patients with circulatory problems in the head following 20 chelation drips.[15] In another study Richard Casdorph treated four patients who were suffering from gangrene in their feet or toes. All of these people had been advised to have amputations below the knee, the routine treatment. In all four cases the gangrene healed up during chelation therapy and the legs were saved. Dramatic before-and-after pictures were included in the article.[16]

In another of Casdorph's studies ejection fractions (heart pumping efficiency) improved in 18 patients by an average of 5 points after 20 chelation drips.[17] This may be the only study published anywhere using any treatment method in which ejection fractions have improved.

Individual case reports describe total clearing of obstructions from arteries with chelation therapy. One physician has a series of ultrasound pictures of his own carotid artery (in the neck). A partial obstruction that had produced stroke-like symptoms dissolved gradually as he received over 100 chelation treatments. Another female patient had an 85 percent obstruction of a carotid artery (neck) open completely and disappear following 60 chelation treatments. The speed of improvement surprised even her chelating doctor.

None of these studies were double-blinded. However it is not necessary to double-blind every study. Double-blind studies are most suitable for drug-versus-placebo types of investigations in which the benefits of the treatment may be small. Many treatments can't be double-blinded because it would be impossible to prevent a patient from knowing he was receiving a treatment or not (i.e., bypass surgery). Also, if results are seen from a treatment that are so spectacular they absolutely never occur with normal care, then insistence on a double-blind study is out of line.

DEATHS FROM CHELATION THERAPY?

In early experimental phases of the study of EDTA in the 1950s, university researchers were giving 10 grams of the drug as a rapid intravenous push. No pre-treatment kidney function tests were performed and nobody was aware some peoples' kidneys may be sensitive to EDTA. Although published reports are lacking, possibly four or six people died during these early high dose experiments. These horrible experiences led to changes in administration of the drug in which much less is given over several hours. Opponents of chelation therapy frequently refer to these deaths now.

Over the years chelation therapy has had a remarkable record for safety. Over 500,000 people have received chelation therapy without a single fatality that has been directly related to the treatment, as long as the ACAM protocol has been followed.

The recommended dose for lead poisoning is now 50 mg per Kg body weight and that is the dose currently recommended for chelation therapy. Chelating physicians usually use 3 grams of EDTA in a 500cc bottle of fluid, and run the drip about three hours. Magnesium (300 mg), vitamin C, potassium, and other nutrients may be added to the bottle as well.

FDA APPROVED STUDY OF CHELATION THERAPY

The FDA approved an Investigational New Drug application (IND) and protocol in 1986 for a double blind controlled study of EDTA chelation therapy. To be eligible to be in the study patients must have arterial insufficiency in the legs (claudication).

Initial studies were scheduled to began in three army hospitals. Plans were made to expand the studies into 20 private hospitals in 1991 when a major drug company offered additional funding. However, the chief of research of the drug company was replaced by a physician who was not receptive to the study and the company's financial commitment was quickly canceled. The study went into limbo pending future funding.

When the Food and Drug Administration approved the application for the study, it did not require phase I (safety) studies. The FDA has known all about EDTA for many years. In its letter approving the study, the FDA wrote that *safety was not an issue.*

Many patients of mine, especially from Alberta, Canada, have told me their doctors have blasted chelation therapy. Some have said goodbye to them because they "were going to take chelation therapy and die." Doctors who terrify potential chelation patients in this manner should be reminded of an interesting fact. When donor hearts for transplant surgery are moved from one city to another by airplane in little coolers, they are immersed in a 100 percent solution of EDTA.

After the FDA study began, the agency's bias against the therapy surfaced. *The FDA Consumer* magazine ran an article on ten remedies it called quackery. The list included EDTA chelation therapy and people were advised to avoid it. Representatives from the organization sponsoring the study (ACAM) contacted the FDA about this outrageous action. It was highly inappropriate for one department of the FDA to attack a treatment while it was under investigation by a different department. A later issue of *FDA Consumer* carried both a retraction and a apology.

The *New England Journal of Medicine* published another example of bias against EDTA. After quantitative angiography, doctors advised a 55-year-old man to have bypass surgery. The man chose to take chelation therapy instead. No mention was made if his symptoms improved with the therapy or not.

When his symptoms became worse one year later, he returned to the medical center and the quantitative angiogram was repeated. The authors stated obstructions increased in one artery. However, before-and-after photographs were printed in the article which showed many other arteries had opened up. In any event, on the basis of this one case, the authors concluded EDTA chelation therapy was an unacceptable therapy for coronary disease.[18]

Political battles over chelation therapy continue to rage. Some state medical licensing boards continue to bring disciplinary actions against chelation physicians. Others have tried to make the treatment illegal. This has happened in California, Indiana, Arizona (the Osteopathic board) and West Virginia.

Chelation therapy does not work all the time. Nothing does. I have been using the treatment since 1984 and have seen very good results in a high percentage of patients. Some of these patients' doctors had told them they were too sick to have any kind of surgery.

My most dramatic chelation result has been in a man who was advised to have a heart transplant at the age of 47. He went on a natural food diet, multivitamin/mineral supplements, took chelation treatments and is alive and functioning now, six years later.

Chelation doctors don't just hook up the bottles and let them drip. They encourage patients to follow lower fat diets of fresh, unprocessed, unrefined foods, take nutritional supplements, get modest exercise, practice stress reduction, and stop smoking. The combination creates a powerful healing effect in most people. Many patients can avoid balloon jobs and cabbages with this approach. Chelation can bring about improvements bypass surgery and efforts to simply reduce cholesterol can't match.

Opponents of chelation therapy continue to denounce the treatment. If patients say they have improved after chelation therapy most doctors say that this is all in their heads and represents nothing more than the action of a placebo. If this is so, then chelation therapy is one of the best placebos ever found. Other placebos should work so well.

TOTAL PARENTERAL NUTRITION (TPN)

In the early 1970s Dr. Stanley Dudrick of Houston, Texas, pioneered the development of total parenteral nutrition. This is the process of feeding people through the vein. The intravenous mixture contains all of the amino acids, vitamins, minerals, essential fatty acids and trace minerals a person needs to survive. This has been a lifesaving procedure for many people who can't take nutrients by mouth for a variety of reasons such as surgical removal of most of the intestines, obstructions due to adhesions, or being born with no intestines.

Over the years some patients who had been on intravenous feedings died in accidents. Some of these people were known to have previous coronary artery disease, but at autopsy their arteries were found to have improved. This attracted Dr. Dudrick's attention.

Dudrick was a cabbage surgeon by training. He says that when he was doing bypasses he began to think about the disease process involved in coronary artery disease. He realized the disease was progressing along right under his fingertips while he was tying the bypass veins in place.

This led to several years of rabbit studies in which he induced atherosclerosis with diets. Then he suspended the rabbits in the air with slings so they couldn't move, and gave them intravenous feeding (TPN). Dudrick tried many formulas. The only one that cleaned out the arteries was an amino acid mixture patterned after the composition of a vegetarian diet.

Before Dudrick was ready to move on to trying the method in humans, he was talked into treating some desperately ill people. His first case was a man whose angina was so bad he couldn't get out of bed to go to the bathroom. Within weeks of beginning the special TPN mixture the man flew from his home in Boston to Florida and went deep sea fishing.

Dudrick progressed on to study 35 atherosclerotic patients. After three months on the special TPN drips all 35 showed plaque regression in the aorta, the carotid (neck), and iliac (groin) arteries. The patients had improved blood flow, improved ejection fractions of the ventricles of the heart, and improved ventricular wall motion.[19]

The method is complicated, cumbersome and expensive. People treated this way need to have an indwelling catheter implanted surgically and receive an intravenous drip sixteen hours a day, every day. The therapy runs for six to nine months at a cost of over $30,000. During this time the only thing patients are allowed to take by mouth is water.

After these successes, Dudrick fed the rabbits orally the same intravenous mixture that had worked well intravenously. These efforts were unsuccessful. Apparently the gastrointestinal tract did something to block any favorable action. The method has received little publicity, but it does prove once again that the body is able to reverse atherosclerosis.

There is one principle we can learn from the effective methods described in this chapter. Our bodies have a wonderful ability to heal themselves. We apparently bring arterial disease upon ourselves through a combination of poor diets and lifestyles. However, it now has been proven to the satisfaction of the biggest skeptics in medicine that our arteries have the ability to heal and dissolve away fatty obstructions.

WHY DO THESE THERAPIES WORK?

There is no simple answer to this question. Some answers are offered, but the problem is complex. Studies in primitive lifestyle people show that when humans live in an environment with clean air, clean water, and eat fresh wholesome food, they can remain free of coronary artery disease and other degenerative diseases.

An old cat feeding study from the 1940s demonstrated this relationship. Cats fed a diet of 100 percent raw food stayed healthy through several generations. Other cats were fed the same food, but parts of it were cooked. Those cats began to experience diseases of physical degeneration and the degree of the problems increased with each succeeding generation. One third generation cat that experienced severe physical degenerative changes did recover to a state of good health after escaping the living nearby in the wild (on mice, etc.).[20]

This pattern resembles what is being seen in humans. This study has never been repeated or analyzed to try to explain how the heart treatment altered the food in such a negative way.

Pritikin and Ornish both were believers in the cholesterol theory. Both believed if a reduction of dietary fat from 40 to below 30 percent (the American Heart Association recommendation) doesn't work, then people should drop their fat intake down to the level of total vegetarians. Both used diets of no greater than 10 percent fat, and both programs worked. Ornish has been able to present his study at conventional medical meetings because the results sound like they are related to the *politically correct* cholesterol theory.

However, people can't go on a 10 percent fat diet without making other drastic changes in their food consumption, and these are never mentioned. To make up for a reduction in fat calories, people must consume much larger quantities of fresh vegetables, fruits, and whole grains. When people substitute complex carbohydrates for simple carbohydrates, fresh vegetables for commercially canned and frozen, and reduce sugar intake drastically, the intake of vitamins and minerals and other antioxidants may go up four to six-fold. As you will see later, this can make all the difference in the world.

When a person decides to become a vegetarian he unknowingly changes his nutritional intake in this manner. He reduces his intake of fats while he increases his intake of nutrients that help our biochemistry process fats efficiently. Therefore, a lot more is going on than simply a reduction in fat.

I believe it is very *unlikely* that fat reduction by itself contributes much to improvement. The American Heart Association does not advise changes in the remainder of the diet. People who follow the AHA diet usually continue to consume junk food and refined carbohydrates, and the coronary artery disease process marches on.

In the case of Dr. G. a program was initiated that included diet and lifestyle changes, in addition to chelation therapy in the early phase. His angina pains went away after taking 20 chelation treatments and he never took any more. Other parts of his program have been keeping him well for the past 25 years.

Dr. G. made dietary changes similar to those described above. He increased his intake of dietary fiber and essential nutrients while he liberally saturated his body with antioxidants in the form of supplements. He was years ahead of recommendations that are beginning to flow from the new oxidation theory of arterial wall damage.

TRADITIONAL CHINESE MEDICINE

Western medical philosophy is oriented around dissecting a problem into tiny pieces, then launching a direct frontal attack on a small part of the problem. Researchers developed a belief system that preached that high blood cholesterol levels caused atherosclerosis. Therefore, the logical action would be to try to bring blood cholesterol levels down at all cost, even if the treatment ends up increasing overall death rates. If a coronary artery is partially blocked, clean it out, bypass it, stretch it, scrape it out, burn it out with a laser. Call in the plumbers.

The basic concept of traditional Chinese medicine couldn't be more different. The Chinese believe a subtle energy system functions in the body that maintains balance and harmony. It is this energy system that regulates our biochemistry. In contrast, Western medicine offers no explanation at all for what orchestrates our biochemistry and any efforts to investigate electromagnetic phenomena in the body are resisted.

According to the Chinese, if this energy system is in good balance we stay well. We become ill only when our energy system is out of balance. The Chinese say we upset this system in our bodies with poor diets, lack of exercise, stress, pollution, excess alcohol, and a host of other poor health habits. This begins to sound vaguely familiar.

Therefore, fatty obstructions grow in arterial walls because the subtle energy system has gotten out of balance. The body can dissolve fatty obstructions in arterial walls, but only when a state of normal balance has been reestablished. This would explain how the fatty obstructions in Ornish's study opened 8.6 percent in one year without drugs or surgery. The patients' own healing efforts kicked in and dissolved them.

The Pritikin Program and chelation therapy programs must be working the same way. The only way to get rid of fatty obstructions throughout the arterial system is to do what is necessary to get back into normal balance so the body will try to heal itself. Western medicine views this entire concept as wild, strange, and unproven.

All of the many therapies of traditional Chinese medicine are intended to improve this energy balance. The system of traditional Chinese medicine is immense and complicated, developed over a period of 4,000 years. The Chinese never tried to prove effectiveness of these therapies scientifically until about 1980. Since that time much of what remained mere theory for 3,000 years has now been proven in sophisticated tests using modern high technology methods. Unfortunately, few Westerners are aware of these studies.

BALANCE IN THE BODY AND TOOTH DECAY

This concept of subtle mechanisms and balance was studied many years ago in the area of tooth decay. Primitive lifestyle people remained almost free of tooth decay, though they practiced no more dental hygiene than picking food from between their teeth with twigs. They also didn't take fluoride treatments, or add fluoride to their water. However, as soon as they began to consume the foods of modern commerce, oral problems of many kinds began to appear.

Ralph Steinman, D.D.S., of Loma Linda Dental School, worked for many years on the study of fluid flow through teeth. When a person or animal is in good health the flow goes from the inside of the tooth to the outside. This helps wash off food particles that might cling to teeth. When we are ill, in poor energy balance, or have eaten junk food, the fluid flow reverses and goes from the outside of the tooth to the inside. This direction of the flow helps food particles stick to the surfaces of teeth and set us up for tooth decay.

Most people can experience this phenomena themselves. If they eat only fresh natural foods for several days and floss and brush as usual at bedtime, teeth feel clean to the tongue upon awakening. If they eat some pie or cake for dinner, the next morning the tongue can usually detect a white film on the teeth which can be scraped off with a fingernail. Try this out some time.

Steinman worked out these relationships in small animals using dyes to detect which way the fluid flow was going. In one of his most disturbing experiments he fed weanling rats solutions of refined sugar, but stopped feeding the sugar a few days before any teeth erupted. When the teeth came in they decayed away although they had never been in direct contact with sugar. it is most likely the explanation for this phenomena relates to a disruption of energy balance throughout the body as postulated in traditional Chinese medicine.[21]

SUMMARY

Ample evidence now exists that the body can heal and dissolve away obstructions in coronary arteries without drugs. Programs that accomplish this involve major diet and lifestyle changes. For these improvements to occur, conditions must exist that allow the body's healing mechanisms to kick in and function. In the final analysis, it is the body that must do the healing by improving the biochemical function in our tissues and absorbing fatty obstructions.

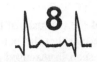

8

NUTRIENT CONNECTIONS

Eat as if your life depended on it.
Anonymous

In contrast to the weak associations between cholesterol, fats, and coronary artery disease, other nutritional associations are very strong. These findings have been almost totally ignored because the cholesterol theory has dominated the subject so completely.

Prior to the advent of the cholesterol theory, most doctors assumed that our bodies could run perfectly well on any kind of food we decided to pour into our stomachs. When I was in medical school in the late 1950s we did not receive one hour of instruction in nutrition with the exception of learning about diets for diabetics. We would never dream of approaching maintenance of our cars with a similar cavalier philosophy. Intuition tells us that if we supply our cars with high quality oil, gasoline, and keep engines in tune, they will purr along for many extra years. Our bodies should be so lucky.

EXPERIMENTAL ATHEROSCLEROSIS FROM HIGH-FAT DIETS

Atherosclerosis can be induced in animals, but the way in which researchers accomplish this should cause concern. A commonly used atherogenic diet for rabbits consists of 10 percent saturated fat, 10 percent corn oil, and high amounts of vitamin D-3. This diet sounds similar to what a typical American teenager may consume who drinks a lot of vitamin D-3 fortified milk. It also doesn't sound too much different from the diet recommended by the American Heart Association.

In many studies animals have been placed on diets that are very strange for them. A logical person would expect animals in such experiments to not do well on these diets, and that is what is seen. An example is the feeding of high fat foods to vegetarian rabbits. However, when such a study yields results that support a prevailing dogma, researchers have shown no restraint in making the giant leap of extrapolating the results to humans.

When vegetarian rabbits eat a diet that is high in saturated fats and cholesterol, they develop a form of atherosclerosis that may totally plug up their coronary arteries within three months. Supporters of the cholesterol theory have used this observation to support the theory, ignoring the fact that the pathological changes in the animals' arteries in no way resemble those seen in diseased arteries of humans. In vegetarian animals the fatty deposits build up on the inner walls of arteries. In humans, the fatty deposits grow *within* the arterial wall itself and are covered by the inner lining membrane of the artery. In any event, the ability to produce fatty deposits in arteries in animals made it possible to study the effect of the manipulation of nutrients on the fatty deposits.

In one study animals were fed an atherogenic diet but were also given eight times the recommended intake of magnesium. No fatty deposits formed. When the study was repeated with lower levels of magnesium, plus some vitamin B-6, the animals also were protected from atherosclerosis.

If animal handlers protect dietary fats from becoming oxidized from the air, the animals can eat a high-fat diet and remain free of coronary artery disease without taking the supplements. No fatty obstructions form, though blood cholesterol levels may go as high as 2,000 mg/dl, ten times the upper limit currently considered acceptable for humans.

In the 1970s researchers discovered dietary cholesterol existed in two forms, *oxidized* and *reduced*. In fresh, natural foods, cholesterol and fats occur only in the harmless reduced form. Only the oxidized form is toxic to arteries (see Chapter 9). A fat becomes oxidized when some of its hydrogen atoms have been replaced with oxygen or oxygen compounds. The common term for this change is to say that a fat has gone rancid.

The 1911 rabbit experiments that launched the cholesterol theory were reexamined from this viewpoint. As expected, it was discovered handlers had done the most expedient thing. They had simply plopped the high fat food into cages once a day. This allowed fat molecules on the surface of the blob of food to react with oxygen from the air and become oxidized.

Some researchers were curious enough to repeat the original rabbit feeding studies. They fed one group of rabbits a diet containing 1 percent oxidized cholesterol and the animals developed extensive obstructions in their coronary arteries. A second group ate the same amount of fat and cholesterol, but care was taken to protect the food from oxidation. Arteries in those rabbits remained disease free.

NUTRITIONAL DEFICIENCIES
AND CORONARY ARTERY DISEASE

Some animal species have developed coronary artery disease on diets which were manipulated to be deficient in a single nutrient. This result has been seen in studies with magnesium, vitamin B-6, zinc, selenium, copper, and chromium.

In efforts to keep scientific studies simple, nutrition studies usually manipulate only one nutrient at a time. I am not aware of any studies in which researchers have produced borderline deficiencies of several nutrients simultaneously, as must frequently occur in the typical American diet.

The late Dr. Roger Williams was well qualified to inform the public about nutrition. He was professor of chemistry at the University of Texas, founder of the Clayton Foundation (where many vitamins were discovered), and sat on the board that set the first minimum daily allowances. He discovered pantothenic acid and named folic acid. Williams wrote several books for the lay public when he was in his 90s including *Nutrition Against Disease*.[1] That book contains 124 pages of references and abstracts of papers documenting nutrient-disease relationships.

For example, monkeys fed a vitamin B-6 deficient diet develop atherosclerosis rapidly.[2] A mechanism for this observation exists which involves the biochemistry of homocysteine. In another example, oral zinc supplements were found to significantly inhibit the formation of atherosclerotic plaques in rabbits that were fed a high cholesterol diet.[3]

Dr. Williams expressed a concern about people worrying unnecessarily about their cholesterol levels. He believed that if someone consumes a wide assortment of wholesome foods that provide all of the essential nutrients, amounts adequate to run our biochemistry smoothly, then serum cholesterol will take care of itself and we don't need to worry about it.[4]

HUMAN STUDIES

Researchers have studied nutritional relationships with coronary artery disease in various ways. Sections of diseased arteries have been found to contain lower levels of trace minerals than arteries from people who died in accidents.[5] heart attack patients usually have lower than normal levels of zinc in their plasma.[6] In one study 18 of 24 patients with severe symptomatic atherosclerosis improved markedly when they were placed on high dose zinc sulfate pills three times a day for one year.[7]

VITAMIN B-6

Vitamin B-6 (pyridoxine) deficiency is common in heart disease patients. Vitamin B-6 status can be determined by a biochemical challenge test. When a person is deficient in vitamin B-6, an oral load of the amino acid tryptophan will produce an increased spill of xanthurenic acid in the urine. Scientists accept this test as a reliable measure of B-6 needs in the body.[8] Because of results of this test, Roger Williams speculated that patients with coronary artery disease have higher than average requirements for vitamin B-6 because of their individual genetic patterns.

MAGNESIUM

Magnesium is the most prevalent trace mineral in the body, the catalyst for several hundred intracellular enzymes. This single mineral has attracted so much attention that a yearly international conference is held to discuss new studies on magnesium alone. Many studies have linked magnesium deficiency to coronary artery disease.

If rats consume magnesium supplements before researchers tie off their left main coronary arteries, heart attacks do not occur. Adequate levels of magnesium inhibit the stickiness of platelets. Magnesium plays a pivotal role in energy metabolism. Geographic areas with soft water (low mineral content) have been found to have higher rates of coronary artery disease. [9, 10]

Mineral levels of the ashes of people who have died of arterial spasm have been measured. Tissue levels of magnesium were 15 to 30 percent lower than those of matched controls who died of other causes. This led investigators to study the relationship between magnesium and coronary artery spasm. Five different animal species were used in the studies. In all of the species tested, as body levels of magnesium decreased, the amount of coronary artery spasm increased.[11]

Human magnesium studies continue to grow in number, and some progressive hospitals now use the mineral in the treatment of heart attack patients. A study in one hospital involved two groups each containing 100 heart attack patients. On admission, one group received a placebo shot, the other an injection of magnesium sulfate. There were two deaths among those who received the magnesium, seven in the placebo group. Researchers concluded that the magnesium administration reduced both the incidence of serious abnormal rhythms of the heart as well as coronary artery spasm.[12]

A British study confirmed these results. Acute heart attack patients who received magnesium by slow intravenous drip had an in-hospital death rate of only 7 percent. In the group that did not receive magnesium the death rate was 19 percent.[13]

In another study, 100 patients admitted with heart attacks received intramuscular injections of magnesium sulfate every day for 12 days. Only one death occurred which was attributable to coronary artery disease. During the previous year, when magnesium injections had not been used, 30 percent of 196 consecutive patients admitted with heart attacks died.[14]

A *meta-analysis* of magnesium in myocardial infarction (heart attacks) appeared in the American Heart Association's journal, *Circulation*, in 1992. In a meta-analysis statistics are combined from many compatible studies that meet certain criteria. The authors stated that "magnesium is cheap, easy to handle, and relatively free of side effects. Its mechanism may lie in the preservation of myocardium (heart muscle), in addition to arrhythmia suppression. It is at the very least a reasonable form of therapy in acute myocardial infarction."

In this meta-analysis 930 patients were admitted with heart attacks. Administration of intravenous magnesium was associated with a 49 percent reduction in ventricular tachycardia and fibrillation. Overall, there was a 54 percent reduction in mortality.[15]

As promising as these findings are, most hospitals do not yet use magnesium in this way. The magnesium is available in every hospital's obstetrics department where it is used to treat eclampsia, one of the worst complications of pregnancy. But it doesn't seem to make its way to the emergency department and coronary care unit. Most physicians have never studied nutrition, or had any interest in nutritional therapies. Most of their contacts with nutrition have been confrontational with patients who have begun to take an interest in the subject. Patients who are informed in nutrition can't understand why medicine ignores what might be accomplished with nutritional therapies.

These studies on magnesium have appeared in respected medical journals, but it is unlikely many doctors read them. Usually, doctors ignore articles on subjects that sound strange to them.

MEASURING MAGNESIUM LEVELS

Magnesium is not distributed evenly between cells of the body and liquids of the body. The level of magnesium inside cells of our bodies is about 10,000 times higher than outside of cells (in the serum, or liquid part of the blood). As with potassium, when there is a magnesium deficiency, the body makes a serious effort to maintain normal serum levels by shifting more out of cells. Cell levels may fall as much as 30 percent before serum levels begin to fall below the normal range.

When physicians do begin to take an interest in magnesium, their first response usually is to order a *blood* magnesium, or a *serum* magnesium test. Either of these orders directs the laboratory to measure levels in the serum of the blood, the liquid part. Serum magnesium tests may seriously underestimate the true incidence of magnesium deficiency.

A better place to measure magnesium is in a tissue sample such as white and red blood cells which are easy to obtain. These tests are readily available, but when ordered doctors must be specific to avoid confusion with serum tests. To get cell levels blood samples can be drawn locally and sent to special *reference* laboratories that run tests that are less frequently ordered.

On several occasions I have advised a Canadian patient to have a red cell magnesium test ordered by his or her local physician across the border where my request for a lab test would not be honored. Without exception the doctor has ordered a serum test and told the patient it is just as reliable as a cell test.

A study from the University of Southern California exemplifies this difference. Researchers measured magnesium both ways in 100 consecutive patients admitted with heart attacks. Serum magnesium was low in 5 percent of patients. When magnesium was measured in white blood cells from the same samples, 53 percent had low levels.[16]

The most accurate test for magnesium deficiency is more difficult to perform. A known amount of magnesium is given slowly by intravenous drip and urine is collected for several hours. If the body retains more than a certain percentage of the magnesium given, then the patient is deficient.[17] This test occasionally identifies people whose kidneys lose excess amounts of magnesium, which can be another cause of chronic deficiency.

Because excess amounts of oral magnesium have a cathartic effect (Epsom salt used for constipation is magnesium sulfate) it is difficult to build up body stores orally when someone is deficient. Sometimes several intramuscular shots of magnesium sulfate must be given to reach the point where balance can be maintained with oral intake alone.

Why does the average person become deficient in magnesium? According to Dr. Heikki Karppanen, of the University of Helsinki, the dietary intake of magnesium in developed countries has fallen by two thirds in the past 50 years. He used white flour as a prominent example of a reduction of magnesium levels in food. People who eat white flour bread consume only 18 percent of the magnesium they would receive if they ate whole wheat bread. Losses from brown rice to white rice are similar.

Another big drop in intake occurs when people eat commercially canned and frozen vegetables. Up to 50 percent of minerals may leach out during excessive soaking in water at the factory to remove dirt. If these products are then cooked in water and the water is discarded, another 25 percent reduction may occur.

VITAMIN E

About 40 years ago two physicians by the name of Shute wrote several books about the beneficial uses of vitamin E. The medical profession ridiculed them, but their vindication may be at hand. At the time no one considered vitamin E to be an essential nutrient in humans because test subjects placed on vitamin E deficient diets for several years showed no signs of any illness.

Because of this, nutritionists referred to vitamin E as a *vitamin in search of a disease*. This negative attitude is changing and disparaging remarks about vitamin E are no longer heard. Many diseases are now linked to cellular damage from oxidation reactions and vitamin E acts as a powerful antioxidant in the body.

The World Health Organization conducted a study that compared death rates from coronary artery disease with several well accepted risk factors. The association between elevated blood cholesterol, or blood pressure, and coronary artery disease death rates was minimal. The best predictor of heart attack risk turned out to be a low blood level of vitamin E, and the lower the level the greater the risk. The authors concluded, "The differences in coronary artery disease mortality are primarily attributable to plasma status of vitamin E, which might have a protective function."[18]

BETA-CAROTENE

Beta-carotene is the material that gives carrots their characteristic color. The body can convert beta-carotene into vitamin A, but will only do so according to its needs. Because of this relationship, beta-carotene is accepted as being virtually nontoxic. It is also an efficient antioxidant.

Several years ago a number of studies suggested increased consumption of beta-carotene might reduce the incidence of cancer. Harvard Medical School initiated a large study of the preventive effects of aspirin in heart disease and beta-carotene in cancer. A total of 22,000 physicians were recruited as volunteers. In a sub group of doctors with preexisting coronary artery disease, half took supplements of beta-carotene, 50 mg every two days (9 mg equals 15,000 I.U.), and half took a placebo. The study lasted 10 years.

Researchers were disappointed to find no difference in the rate of cancer between the beta-carotene and placebo groups. However, something unexpected happened in the sub-group of doctors with a history of coronary artery disease. Physicians who took beta-carotene experienced a 50 percent reduction in all major cardiovascular events, such as heart attacks, strokes, bypass surgery, or cardiovascular death. The authors said the results suggest that "beta-carotene, a therapy without clinically important side effects, may reduce risks of subsequent vascular events."[19]

This report was published in the medical journal, *Circulation*, which is published by the American Heart Association, the powerful group that has backed the cholesterol theory to the hilt. *Circulation* published the report as a small abstract with the misleading title, "Beta-Carotene Therapy for Chronic Stable Angina." Instead of presenting the findings as an important discovery, the abstract occupied a total page space of only eight square inches. Fortunately, some heart researchers noticed the abstract and publicized the results.

Such a reduction in heart deaths puts efforts based on the cholesterol theory to shame. Researchers stumbled backwards into a therapy that cut heart attack deaths in half with a safe, simple, unpatentable, inexpensive nutritional supplement. These results also eclipse the most optimistic claims of cabbage surgeons and balloon passing cardiologists. If cabbages could be shown to increase the life expectancy of recipients even a little bit, we would never hear the end of it.

VITAMIN C

Many studies show a relationship between vitamin C and atherosclerosis. Deficiencies of vitamin C lead to atherosclerosis in animals, whereas supplementation with vitamin C can cure experimentally produced atherosclerosis. Vitamin C supplementation also reduces the stickiness of platelets, another favorable laboratory indicator.

One study of vitamin C in humans almost came to a tragic end. Human volunteers who consumed a vitamin C deficient diet for several months ran into serious complications that caused a termination of the study. Some suddenly developed cardiac emergencies before any signs of scurvy became obvious.[20] For this reason scientists say that they don't understand the many ways in which the body uses vitamin C. Most of it just seems to disappear into the biochemical machinery of the body.

A recent study reported that older men who consumed 300 to 600 mg a day of vitamin C in pill form for 10 years lived six years longer than those who consumed amounts closer to the Recommended Dietary Allowance. Women with higher intake of vitamin C lived one year longer. This improvement in life expectancy of men almost closes the gap between the sexes.[21] Some people have said that people who believe in taking vitamin pills are probably doing other health supporting things as well, and this could well figure into the results in this study. Ordinary researchers don't seem to be able to figure out what those steps might be because of preexisting biases.

These results are consistent with the oxidation theory of atherosclerosis which is described in the next chapter. Vitamin C is a powerful antioxidant that protects us form oxidized lipoproteins, oxidized polyunsaturated fatty acids, as well as free radicals. [22] (Free radicals are atoms that have an unpaired electron in an outer orbit. They are highly reactive and can do a lot of damage in a short time. They are kept under control in the body by specific enzymes, as well as antioxidant free-radical scavengers such as vitamin C, vitamin E, beta-carotene, selenium based compounds, and others.)

The possible addition of six years to the life expectancy of older men because they did one simple thing caused a stir in the media for only one day. If similar results were seen following drug treatment for elevated blood cholesterol levels, drug companies would announce them widely. Visits by detail men to doctors' offices would increase until almost every man, woman and child had a prescription for the wonder drug in his hand.

A study published in 1960 is of interest here because of its spectacular outcome and its misinterpretation by the author and the journal in which it was published. Lester Morrison put 50 patients with proven coronary artery disease on a low fat diet plus vitamin supplements. Twelve years later 38 percent of these people were still alive. In a control group that stayed on routine diets and did not take supplements, all patients were dead within 12 years. Morrison credited the low fat diet for the increase in survival in the first group.[23]

Because no subsequent low fat diet study has ever shown positive results, the explanation must lie elsewhere. In his low fat diet group, Morrison reported that patients were consuming 140 mg a day of vitamin C in their food. The supplements were said to double this intake to 280 mg per day.

In light of recent studies with vitamin C it appears that the increased levels of this antioxidant were responsible for the increased survival rate, not the low fat diet. If Morrison had been astute enough to reach this conclusion and had given credit to the vitamin C, it is unlikely editors of the conservative *Journal of the American Medical Association* would have accepted the study for publication. The information would have been lost and not sit on medical library shelves today.

The problem with vitamin C is that it's cheap and drug companies can't patent or control it. Therefore, doctors continue to hear about cholesterol-lowering drugs directly from drug company sales people and in advertisements in medical journals, not about vitamin C. No one benefits financially from informing them about the benefits of increased consumption of antioxidants such as vitamin C or beta-carotene. Information about these worthwhile materials dies in libraries along side other useful nutritional therapies.

SALES OF VITAMINS

Factory production of vitamin C increased from 10 million pounds in 1966 to more than 20 million pounds in 1974. Assuming there were about 200,000,000 Americans in 1974, this means each person was consuming an average of 123 mg of supplemental vitamin C daily, in addition to an average dietary intake of about 100 mg. In actual practice, some people must have been consuming more, some a lot less. During this time period the death rate from coronary artery disease began its rapid fall.[24] It is highly probable that increased consumption of vitamin C played a role in this reduction of deaths from the disease, the same as it appears to have done in Morrison's study.

In recent years, Americans have been increasing their consumption of all vitamins. According to the U.S. Department of Commerce, vitamin sales at the

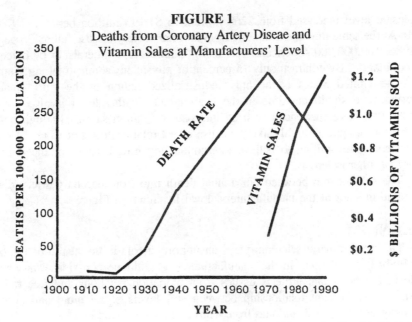

FIGURE 1
Deaths from Coronary Artery Diseae and
Vitamin Sales at Manufacturers' Level

Source: U.S. Department of Commerce and the National Center for Health Statistics.
Vitamin sales went up 4.4 times while the death rate from coronary artery disease
fell by 35 percent.

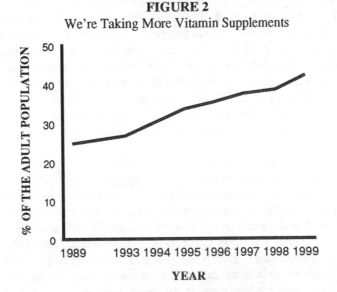

FIGURE 2
We're Taking More Vitamin Supplements

Thirty years ago, few people took vitamin supplements. Today 42 percent of U.S.
adults report that they takes vitamins every day. Source: Multi-Sponsor Surverys Inc,
Princeton, New Jersey, Using Gallup Poll data.

wholesale level increased from $268 million to $1,193 million between 1970 and 1990. At the same time the death rate from coronary artery disease fell by 35 percent. In 1986, 169,000,000 Americans were using vitamins and minerals, or 67 percent of the population. By contrast, only 15 percent of physicians admit to taking vitamins.

The United States is the only industrialized nation in the world that has experienced a significant drop in the heart attack death rate. It is also the only country that has experienced such an increase in vitamin sales. Although only an association, it appears highly likely a cause-effect relationship is at work. More and more people are willing to believe this connection now because of the oxidative theory of atherosclerosis.

The relationship between our annual death rate from coronary artery disease and vitamin sales at the manufacturers' level is shown in Figure 1.

SELENIUM

The trace mineral selenium plays an important role in the health of the heart. The body uses selenium in the manufacture of glutathione peroxidase, an enzyme made in the body that protects tissues from oxidation reactions and free radicals. There is a significant relationship between soil levels of selenium and coronary artery disease. Higher death rates from heart attacks are found in areas of the United States that have low or absent levels of selenium.[25]

In the Pacific Northwest, soils contain no selenium because of ancient glacial actions. Plants and grasses can grow tall and lush because their metabolism does not require selenium. When horses, cattle, goats, and other large animals eat a selenium deficient diet they may develop a condition called *white muscle disease*. Gray streaks are found running through hearts and other muscles when they are butchered.

White muscle disease strikes young animals in a much more dramatic fashion. Several rancher-patients of mine have lost animals to this disease. They describe how they have released young calves into a new field and watched them run playfully into the new pasture. Then, without warning, one of them has dropped dead. An autopsy revealed the tell tale signs of the deficiency disease. As a preventive measure, ranchers and farmers now give injections of selenium to animals and supplement their diets with vitamins/minerals and trace minerals blocks to lick (replacing the old salt block).

The way in which calves die suddenly from white muscle disease is strikingly similar to how infants die from sudden infant death syndrome (SIDS), a disease of unknown cause. I have never heard of researchers approaching the human disease from this angle. If studies comparing the mineral content of babies who die of sudden infant death syndrome with ash mineral content of babies who die in highway accidents have been done I have not found them. Researchers need to study the status of all minerals in these cases. Such a study would be simple to arrange.

Human selenium deficiency can lead to a cardiomyopathy by the name of Keshan's disease. In a cardiomyopathy the heart fails as a pump, continues to enlarge, and does not respond to medicines normally used to treat heart failure.

Keshan's disease was first seen in some areas of China that have soil deficiencies of selenium. In China the problem was solved by giving people in those areas prophylactic selenium supplements and the disease disappeared. The Chinese are too pragmatic to allow preexisting biases which prevent them form carrying out a logical action. Keshan's disease has been reported in the United States, but it is rare.[26]

CHROMIUM

Chromium concentrations in human tissues decline progressively with age in the United States. In most other parts of the world tissue levels *increase* with age. Refining of grains and the consumption of sugar account for most of our low intake. Sugar not only pushes wholesome foods out of the diet but has been shown to increase the loss of chromium in the urine.

Animals fed chromium deficient diets develop atherosclerosis and diabetes mellitus. Regression of atherosclerotic lesions occurs in rabbits with experimentally induced coronary disease when they receive injections of chromium.

FISH OILS

Another area of interest for researchers in coronary artery disease is in fish oils. Certain Eskimo groups in Greenland have a low death rate from coronary artery disease. In a typical over-simplification, researchers have tried to connect this association with a high consumption of a certain fatty acid found in cold, saltwater fish.

In a small town in the Netherlands, researchers collected information about fish consumption from 852 middle-aged men in 1969. Nutritionists took careful dietary histories from participants and their wives. During 20 years of follow-up, 78 men died of coronary artery disease. The death rate was more than 50 percent lower among those who consumed at least 30 grams of fish per day then among those who did not eat fish. The authors concluded that eating as little as two fish dishes per week may help prevent coronary artery disease.[27]

Ocean fish contain a compound called ecisopentaenoic acid that the body converts into a series of about 30 regulation hormones known as prostaglandins. Some are involved in the mechanisms of inflammation and blood clot formation and have obvious connections to coronary artery disease.

If levels of these prostaglandins do not remain in balance, various kinds of tissue damage can occur. One result of an imbalance in these hormones is the tendency for platelets to want to stick to each other, possibly forming a blood clot in a narrowed artery in the heart.

My first introduction to fatty acids came during a medical meeting in 1976. Dr. Alsoph Corwin, professor emeritus of chemistry at Johns Hopkins University, presented what he called a cooking demonstration. This was highly unusual for a medical meeting. There he stood wearing his apron, looking like a chef on a television cooking program.

Dr. Corwin held up a glass beaker full of vegetable oil which had been collected by the age old technique of crushing vegetable seeds in a press. With the room lights off he exposed the oil to an ultraviolet light in front of a white screen. The screen stayed white.

He then held the beaker of oil over the flame of a bunsen burner, brought it to a boil, and again exposed it to the UV light. A light pink color was projected on the screen. It was obvious something in the oil had changed. Dr. Corwin explained that molecules of fatty acids in the oils had been polymerized by the heat. Polymerization involves changes in chemical bonds.

Unprocessed vegetable oils contain several double bonds between their carbon atoms, all referred to as being in the *cis* configuration. Only *cis* bonds are found in fresh foods. Fatty acid molecules are bent a precise number of degrees at each *cis* bond.

High heat treatment can cause these double bonds to break. Some hook back up the same way. Some flip over 180 degrees and reconnect, forming what are called *trans* bonds. At a *trans* bond the molecule straightens into a new shape. All of the common brands of vegetable oil and salad dressings contain *trans* fatty acids. The processing involves heating the oils in a partial vacuum for 12 hours at 385 degrees Fahrenheit.

Molecules with the *trans* bonds comprise an average of 15 percent of all fatty acids in these oils. In margarine and average of about 35 percent of all of the molecules become *trans* fatty acids, but some brands may run as high as 48 percent. Hydrogenated or partially hydrogenated products contain these abnormal *trans* bonds because the hydrogenation process requires high levels of heat.[28]

The body can't use *trans* fatty acids as essential fatty acids. Not only that, *trans* fatty acids block the common enzyme that starts essential fatty acids down their metabolic pathways into prostaglandin regulation hormones.

Some animal feeding studies have been done to try to measure the results of eating *trans* fatty acids, and mixed results have been seen. In some studies the animals were harmed.

Swine fed a diet containing *trans* fatty acids developed more extensive atherosclerotic damage than those fed beef tallow or butter.[29] In other animal studies diets containing hear treated corn oil were found to produce more atherosclerosis than those containing unheated corn oil.[30]

Little information exists about the possible harm to humans from this change from *cis* to *trans* forms. Jane Heimlich described what happened to one researcher who was working in this area in her book, *What Your Doctor Won't Tell You*. After publishing results which were detrimental to the vegetable oil industry, the researcher found she could not longer get funding to continue her work.[31]

In one recent study, humans consumed known amounts of *trans* isomers of oleic acid. This dietary change increased serum LDL (bad) cholesterol and lowered HDL (good) cholesterol , both regarded to be undesirable changes.[32] In another study men ate either a diet high in saturated fat and cholesterol (the control group) or a low fat diet supplemented with four teaspoons of corn oil per day. After two years blood levels of cholesterol in the corn oil group went down, but he incidence of major cardiac events doubled.[33]

Scientists writing about fatty acids have come to the brink of saying that we should not eat oil products containing *trans* fatty acids, then backed off. The scientific method gets in the way. Not enough studies showing harm to humans exist for scientists to take this step publicly and condemn margarine and common brands of vegetable oil. About the worst thing a scientist can do is to make a commitment to a position prematurely, then be wrong. Until their findings can be backed by tons of research, scientists will say nothing.

OTHER NUTRIENT CONNECTIONS

Deficiencies or excesses of certain nutrients have been associated with coronary artery disease. High dietary intake of fructose (the sweetener form corn) can lead to a deficiency of copper which may increase the risk of coronary artery disease. Vitamin B-6 deficiency has led to abnormal rhythms of the heart in rats.

High levels of some nutrients may increase the risk of coronary artery disease. Excess levels of iron and copper in the body can lead to an increased production of free radicals, which can lead to an increase in oxidative damage. There is new interest in this iron connection. Men who donate blood on a regular basis have been found to have fewer heart attacks.

In women a pattern has been found that heart attacks are rare until after they become menopausal. For many years this lower rate was attributed to the protective effects of estrogen. Now, researchers are beginning to believe the delayed onset of coronary artery disease in women may be due to the monthly loss of blood in the menstrual flow which helps to keep body iron levels in a more optimal range.

Thus, certain nutrients have been shown to protect against atherosclerosis, such as vitamins C, B-6, E, beta-carotene, thiamin, nicotinic acid, biotin, folic acid, pantothenic acid, magnesium, chromium, selenium, copper, essential fatty acids, calcium, silicon, and carnitine. Certain materials appear to have negative effects such as sucrose (refined sugar), other refined carbohydrates, margarine and processed vegetable oils, and high body levels of iron and vitamin D.

More evidence is accumulating in support of one of Dr. Roger Williams' concepts. If *optimal* levels of nutrients exist in the body, then our chemistry will function normally and protect us from most degenerative diseases. Dr. Williams also pointed out how hard it was to try to determine optimal levels. Each of us probably has ordinary requirements for most nutrients, but unusually high requirements for a small number of nutrients. He referred to this as *Biochemical Individuality*, the title of his book on this subject.

There may now be a way to determine what intake levels would be optimal for one individual. A new test is available that provides this information by measuring the uptake of individual nutrients in living white blood cells by measuring DNA synthesis.

A BRIEF HISTORY OF THE SCIENTIFIC
STUDY OF NUTRITION

In the early 1800s, most people in North America lived on farms. They subsisted on diets of fresh natural foods they caught, killed, gathered, or grew themselves.

The first major dietary change was an increased intake in the consumption of refined sugar. Consumption has risen from a mere three pounds per person per year in 1800, to about 125 pounds now, if corn syrup products are included. Some breakfast cereals advertised on television programs for children now contain up to 60 percent refined sugar and really qualify to be called candy. You would never guess the sugar content by their appearances.

About 1880 a new steel milling process was developed that allowed millers to crush wheat more thoroughly. This allowed a more thorough separation of fiber from endosperm when the flour is sifted. Unfortunately, nutrients are distributed unevenly in wheat kernels, most being bound to the fiber portion. The result is that our white flour products contain levels of vitamins and minerals that are about 80 percent lower than in whole wheat flour. This milling change reduced the overall intake of nutrients further.

In the early 1900s canned vegetables appeared followed by frozen foods. Excessive washing and heat treatment further reduced nutrient intake.

About 1920 heat treated (containing *trans* fatty acids) vegetable oils became available. Margarine made its debut about 1935.

Since World War II we have seen an explosive growth of a processed food industry that has given us products that are extruded, emulsified, fabricated, blended, and on and on. Basic staples are now treated as nothing more than raw materials that are fractionated, over heated, and manipulated through the tools of *food engineering*.

THE RDA

Researchers didn't discover and isolate vitamins B-1, B-2, and B-3 until the late 1930s. At the time about 15,000 Americans in the southeastern part of the United States were dying each year from pellagra, a vitamin B-3 deficiency disease. By 1940 researchers found that these deaths were seen in people who were poor and subsisted on refined corn products. The logical action at the time would have been to educate the public about what was going on, then encourage consumption of a variety of whole food products that were consumed in the past.

Instead, the usual *quick fix* was implemented. The Federal Government ordered millers to add B-1, B-2, and B-3 and iron to their refined grains. These were about the only nutrients scientists accepted as being essential at the time, in addition to vitamin C. Though the government took this action over 60 years ago, it has never revised the mandate as more information about nutrients became available.

Therefore, it took scientists over 60 years (1880 to 1940) to begin to identify processing related nutrient losses in food. During this time period our disease pattern shifted toward degenerative illness. Few people suspected the two changes might be causally related.[34]

The scientific field of nutrition developed with a very narrow approach. Scientists studied individual nutrients in relation to the development of obvious vitamin deficiency diseases. Recommended intake levels of nutrients (RDAs) were set at borderline deficiency levels, plus an arbitrary safety factor of about 50 percent. Mainstream nutrition has never shown an interest in the concept of *optimal* levels of intake, levels that would encourage our biochemistry to purr along like a finely tuned engine, not cough and sputter and lead us into diseases of physical degeneration.

As each new nutrient was accepted as being essential to health, a lack of knowledge in the past was demonstrated. It is obvious that vitamin B-6 is essential for health in humans, and always has been. It didn't suddenly become essential to health in 1968 when the Food and Nutrition Board added it to the RDA list. The committee took this action only after several babies had developed convulsions that were found to be caused by a deficiency of the vitamin. Because of its sensitivity to high temperatures vitamin B-6 was being completely destroyed at the factory in the heat sterilization of commercial baby formula. Little babies who were being fed only formula were receiving no B-6 at all.[35]

RDA values became the backbone of the analytic approach in nutrition (versus the anthropological approach). The average run of the mill college level nutrition course stresses these values. If some independent researcher challenges that quality of our modern food supply, defenders of the status quo rally behind the RDA values. They behave as if God carved the levels in stone and the Food and Nutrition Board brought the tablets down from the mountain top as a mandate to the people.

However, many examples exist where nutrient intake levels far above the RDA levels are not only useful but accepted as being necessary. Conventional physicians use *mega* doses of specific vitamins to treat about 40 diseases that are referred to as *inborn errors of metabolism*. Many other examples exist where nutritional supplementation can prevent diseases and help control certain medical problems.[36] Cardiologists are prescribing doses of the niacin form of vitamin B-3 in levels 200 to 300 times the RDA in efforts to reduce blood cholesterol. They try to avoid the stigma of practicing *mega-vitamin therapy* by using the chemical names of the vitamin (niacin and nicotinic acid) and saying they are using pharmacologic doses.

Current RDA levels will sustain life and keep people from dropping dead in the street with an obvious vitamin deficiency disease. However, there is evidence that higher levels, more on a par with those consumed in a primitive diet, would help to prevent coronary artery disease and other diseases of physical degeneration.

Reliance on a numbers approach to nutrition, such as the RDA list, is dangerous. This is its history, and I believe it is naive for us to think we have all the answers in nutrition even now. The only way to be certain we get the nutrients we need to stay healthy is to eat like our ancestors ate as much as possible. It worked for them. People who have remained free of our diseases of physical degeneration had access only to fresh, natural, unprocessed foods.

I like to repeat a story Dr. Jon Wright tells about how far we have come in changing our food supply. A primitive hunter stalks a deer and lets his arrow fly scoring a fatal hit. The hunter runs up to the animal, slits its belly open, plunges his hand into the opening and pulls out a *jelly filled donut*.

Now we have so-called *foods* such as *turkey loaf* which is made of a blend of dehydrated turkey meat, emulsifiers, stabilizers, preservatives, and other strange compounds most people can't even begin to pronounce (an old saying goes, if you can't pronounce it, don't eat it). The gooey blend is extruded from a machine like toothpaste, sliced, wrapped, and sold in stores where it is purchased by the average housewife who has no idea she is buying something far different from natural turkey meat.

We have *instant* potatoes and sugar loaded yogurt. All are purchased with a broad assumption that they are nutritional equivalents of the natural fresh foods. Ice cream is viewed as being nutritious because it has some milk in it, potato chips because they have potatoes in them. Candy bars are advertised as being good for us because they have some nuts in them. The processed food industry has taken a nutritionally ignorant population and confused it further.

Remember that the RDA values are intended to be minimum intake levels needed by healthy people. The Food and Nutrition Board of the National Academy of Sciences itself cautions that different people have individual requirements for nutrients because of differences in genetic make up. They recommend higher intakes during illness and other kinds of stress. That begins to sound like all of us.

DR. PAULING AND THE RDAS

Considering the current state of health in the United States, Dr. Linus Pauling has said that, rather than keeping us in a state of good health, current RDA values are set at levels that will keep us in a state of poor health. He referred to the RDAs as one of the myths of nutrition in a conference in San Francisco in 1978.

Pauling also said he believed the field of nutrition suffered an arrest in its development around 1950. Since that time political positions favoring the processed food industry have taken precedence over new discoveries in the field. Nutritionists have gone along with the positions of the processed food industry and don't seem to realize the importance of their own field in terms of the prevention and treatment of chronic diseases.

What seems to have bothered nutritionists the most was the observation that some individuals were popping vitamins by the handfuls. They recoiled and adopted a position that people should eat a *balanced* (a meaningless term) diet and not take any vitamins as supplements.

Nutritionists frequently repeat their fears that if people take vitamins they will not be as careful about the quality of their food and eat poorly. This fear does not appear to be justified. People I see who take vitamins usually are more concerned about food quality than people who do not take vitamins. At the same time nutritionists stress that we should get all our nutrients from food, they admit that most Americans don't really do well in achieving this goal.

Successful therapies using vitamin and mineral supplements are beginning to appear more frequently in respected journals. Nutritionists continue to ignore the studies and recommend against the use of supplements. Their stance remains the same even in the face of documented reductions in death rates when people have taken higher than dietary levels of beta-carotene, vitamin C, and other antioxidants.

In the 1970s nutritional surveys of Americans conducted by the U.S. Department of Agriculture reported that deficiencies of certain nutrients were widespread. Only a handful of biochemists and nutritionists expressed alarm about these findings. Most nutrition experts looked at the same studies and proudly proclaimed that there was no problem of malnutrition in the average American home, no problem with the average American diet. I believe these conflicts in nutrition have hindered progress in trying to end our coronary artery disease problem.

CONCLUSIONS

A large body of nutritional research exists connecting dietary changes to coronary artery disease. Many of the connections are direct. Experimental deficiency of several specific nutrients has caused coronary artery disease in animals. In many experiments the addition of a specific nutrient has lowered death rates from coronary artery disease in humans. The intravenous infusion of several nutrients has allowed animals to survive surgical obstruction of their left main coronary artery. Results of these experiments are far more impressive than any treatments based on the cholesterol theory.

Recent studies report benefits from the consumption of antioxidants nutrients in humans. In one study men who took beta-carotene had 50 percent fewer heart attack deaths over a 10 year period. In another, increased vitamin C intake appeared to increase life expectancy of older men by as much as six years. A low blood level of vitamin E was found to be the most accurate predictor of heart attack risk in a large European study.

It is my opinion that establishment medicine needs to undergo a paradigm shift in its attitude toward fresh, unprocessed foods as well as nutritional supplements.

9

PREVENT
ARTERIAL "RUST"

You can cure retail but you can only prevent wholesale
Brock Chisholm

Discoveries have appeared during the past 10 years that have led to a new explanation of how fatty obstructions form in artery walls. In humans cholesterol and other fats don't simply come bouncing merrily along down an artery and suddenly decide to stick somewhere. That is what happens when vegetarian animals are fed high fat, high cholesterol diets.

In humans, fatty obstructions are built on location, within the walls of arteries themselves. The process is complicated but mechanisms involved have been worked out so thoroughly it is accepted by the scientific community. Reasonable preventive and treatment actions based on these new findings are effective and simple.

The new theory is called the *oxidation theory*. Oxidation refers to the process of some material combining with oxygen, either in the air or in the body, to form a different compound. Pipes and other metals that have been oxidized are referred to as being rusted. Fats that have become oxidized are referred to as being rancid. Although many specifics of the theory are not yet clear, the framework is in place. A simplified version of the oxidation theory follows.

HOW THE OXIDATION THEORY WORKS

The process begins with some sort of injury to the inner lining of an artery. Cells in the arterial wall immediately below this damaged area begin to actively pick up oxidized lipoprotein (a fat molecule combined with a protein molecule) from the blood. According to experts with strong ties to the cholesterol theory, the main material picked up in arterial walls is oxidized LDL, one of the fractions of cholesterol. Other experts say the material accumulated is not oxidized LDL at all. In any event, there is agreement that only oxidized fats are involved.

Other materials such as cholesteryl esters, calcium, fibrinogen, and other fatty materials, become incorporated in the buildup to form atheromas, or fatty streaks. As these fatty buildups grow and expand they must have some place to go. Arterial walls contain a layer of strong circular muscles. Therefore, the growths have only one way to expand and that is by protruding into the opening of an artery. Over many years the process gradually obstructs an artery, bit by bit (Figure 1).[1]

In the mid 1980s researchers discovered oxidized LDL was toxic to cells, whereas *native* LDL is not.[2] Native LDL is the type of LDL our bodies normally make. Because the peroxidation (oxidation) of LDL was found to be inhibited by antioxidants, an interest developed in the maintenance of adequate tissue levels of antioxidants. This accumulation of oxidized fats can occur only in areas where tissue levels of antioxidants have become depleted. Some of the principle antioxidants in the body are vitamins A, E, and C, as well as beta-carotene and an enzyme which incorporates selenium.

The oxidative theory explains why the old 1911 rabbit feeding experiments came out as they did. The high fat content food sat at room temperature exposed to the air, allowing surface fats to oxidize. That is why when researchers repeated the rabbit experiments in the 1970s, but protected the food from oxidation, the animals' arteries remained healthy. In some feeding studies, rabbits' blood cholesterols went as high as 1,500 to 2,000 mg/dl but no fatty deposits formed.

FIGURE 1

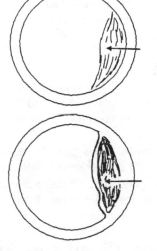

In vegetarian animals fats from the blood stick to the inner walls of arteries.

In humans fatty deposits are built on location within the walls of arteries.

BABOON HAS LAST LAUGH

A patient of mine once told me of an animal feeding study in which he participated. John worked in a regional *primate center*, one of several research centers funded by the Federal Government. One old baboon named George was selected to participate in the study because he had a mean disposition and none of the animal keepers liked him.

The staff dreamed up an experiment in which George was given the opportunity to give his life for science and not be around to bother them any more. They fed the old baboon nothing but hard boiled eggs for one year, then *put him down* (killed him) and performed an autopsy.

Because of the propaganda about the cholesterol theory, the staff confidently expected to find massive obstructions in the old baboon's arteries. They dreamed of seeing their names in large print on the top of a published scientific paper supporting the widely accepted and popular cholesterol theory.

But it was the old baboon who had the last laugh. Because no evidence of atherosclerosis was found in George's arteries, no paper was written. This feeding study demonstrated once again that the fats and cholesterol in fresh eggs are harmless because they have not become oxidized. It also demonstrated that studies that do not support an accepted theory usually don't get published.

The oxidation theory is one reason why people living primitive lifestyles did not experience coronary artery disease. They ate only natural fresh foods. Leftovers were thrown away or fed to animals. Fresh foods from nature do not contain oxidized fats, so these people probably ate very few. Their diets also contained higher levels of antioxidants than are present in the modern industrial food supply.

Many primitive lifestyle people living in the tropics continue to consume 2,000 to 3,000 mg a day of vitamin C each day in their foods. Some people in Fiji were found to be eating as much as 8,000 mg of vitamin C per day in their food. Other cultures that ate grains ate whole grains that still contained full quotas of vitamin E.

The oxidation theory also is consistent with epidemiologic studies connecting high coronary artery disease death rates with selenium deficient soil. Our bodies incorporate selenium into glutathione peroxidase, an enzyme with antioxidant properties.

STUDIES WITH ANTIOXIDANTS

The oxidation theory has stimulated researchers to study the effect of multiple doses of antioxidants on lipid peroxides (oxidized fats) in the blood. This may be the first time that more than one or two nutrients have been used in an experiment at the same time.

At the University of Helsinki 45 nursing home patients received either a placebo or an *antioxidant cocktail*. The cocktail contained vitamins B-6 and C, and the trace minerals zinc and selenium. Test subjects felt better subjectively, serum selenium levels increased, and serum lipid peroxides went down, all desirable responses that would be expected to help prevent fatty deposits from forming in arteries.[3]

In a similar study 80 men received either an antioxidant cocktail or a placebo for five months. People in the study group consumed 600 mg of vitamin C, 300 mg of vitamin E, 27 mg of beta-carotene, and 75 mcg of selenium daily. Oxidation products in the blood went down by 20 percent and the tendency of platelets to stick together (platelet aggregation) went down by 24 percent. Both are desirable changes.[4]

The oxidation theory helps explain why researchers found fewer heart attack deaths in the Harvard sponsored Physicians' Health Study. Physicians who took 50 mg of beta-carotene every second day had half as many fatal heart attacks as doctors in the placebo group over a 10 year period. Beta-carotene is a powerful antioxidant. If the oxidation theory had not been well developed and accepted, it is unlikely the results of this heart study would have been published.

The oxidation theory is consistent with several other research findings from the past. In some studies the incidence of cancer increased as dietary intake of polyunsaturated fats went up. Polyunsaturated fats are subject to becoming oxidized in the body, especially if levels of antioxidants are low. In one recent study in rats, 37 percent of animals fed high levels of corn oil developed cancer of the pancreas compared to only 15 percent of control animals.[5]

Many people link these types of findings to low levels of vitamin E in the average American diet. Several years ago the American Heart Association advised us to increase our intake of polyunsaturated fats, but no accompanying recommendation was made to consume more vitamin E which would have helped to protect from oxidation reactions.

When cancer rates went up the American Heart Association advised us to reduce our intake of polyunsaturated fats from 30 to 10 percent of the diet. This change was made without an explanation. Of course, it would have been awkward to announce publicly that the diet the American Heart Association had been recommending for several years might increase the incidence of cancer.

Several experimental diets have produced atherosclerosis in animals. Most have contained 10 percent corn oil. Some recent studies have intentionally contained oxidized cholesterol as well. Unfortunately, older scientific articles didn't specify if cholesterol or fats in the diets were oxidized or not. If not specified, it is safe to assume that steps were not taken to protect fats from oxidation, usually because researchers did not appreciate the difference at the time.

This raises a question about the validity of all of the old studies in which animals were fed unusually large amounts of fat. Another problem is that most dietary studies don't report intake levels of antioxidants. Therefore, it is safe to assume that most fat feeding studies reported over the past 80 years are worthless.

Other compounds have protective antioxidant activity, such as the amino acid taurine. In one study rabbits ate a 2 percent cholesterol diet for 14 days (probably oxidized as the distinction was not mentioned). One half of the rabbits received supplements of taurine. Animals receiving taurine supplements formed fewer atheromas.[6]

The oxidative theory helps to explain what has been observed in another kind of animal experiment. As mentioned earlier, when the left main coronary artery is tied off abruptly, dogs usually die in less than one hour. However, if researchers inject vitamin E into a vein immediately before tying off the artery, the animals live longer, and some even survive the massive insult. Applying this to humans the expectation would be that people who suffer a heart attack whose tissues contain protective levels of antioxidants should have higher survival rates.

Certainly we are going to hear much more about the oxidative theory in the future. Until it becomes well publicized there are simple protective steps we all can take. We can't afford to wait for years until researchers confirm all aspects of the theory and a recommendation to consume extra antioxidants finally trickles down from ivory towers and the American Heart Association. The step are simple:

1. We can increase our intake of antioxidants right now.

2. We can avoid eating foods that contain oxidized fats (once they are identified).

Medical researchers are cautious about making sweeping recommendations. There are also other barriers in the way of this common sense advice.

For years doctors have been taught that taking vitamin and mineral supplements was a waste of money. Most doctors and nutritionists have told us the food supply is just fine and everything we need to eat to stay healthy is present in our modern supermarket foods. All we need to do is go to the supermarket and buy what we like.

Doctors are not likely to rapidly shift their attitudes 180 degrees and tell us to take pills containing vitamins C, E, A, selenium beta-carotene, etc. This would be on the same order of magnitude as asking them to change religions.

Another problem pertains to existing recommendations concerning what to eat and not to eat. Promoters of the cholesterol theory recommend we avoid eating many natural fresh foods, simply because they have a high saturated fat or cholesterol content. To demonstrate what a ridiculous recommendation this has been, consider this observation. Primitive lifestyle people ate these foods throughout history and did very well on them.

We have been advised to avoid such wholesome fresh foods as eggs, salmon, avacado, crab, lobster, shrimp, and beef. According to the oxidation theory, these foods should cause no problems for us (as in the past) unless they have been mishandled in ways that allow oxidation changes to occur.

Much more dangerous to our health are heat treated vegetable oils and foods containing oxidized fat. These include cake, candy, cookies, pie, pastry, powdered milk, powdered eggs, and many materials commonly used by food processors.

LIPOPROTEIN (a), NEW KID ON THE BLOCK

Lipoprotein (a) closely resembles low density lipoprotein, otherwise known as the LDL fraction of cholesterol (a lipoprotein is nothing more than a fat molecule that is hooked together with a protein molecule). Some researchers say it is lipoprotein (a), not oxidized LDL, that arterial wall cells accumulate and incorporate into fatty growths.

According to Matthias Rath and Linus Pauling, confusion has arisen because, in postmortem examinations of fatty growths in arteries, apolipoprotein (a) splits into apo (a) and LDL-like particles. When improper laboratory methods are used to identify what this fatty material is, it looks like oxidized LDL. According to Rath, when appropriate laboratory methods of analysis are used, the fatty growths can be shown to be composed mostly of lipoprotein (a) and fibrin, not oxidized LDL.[7]

The distribution of blood levels of lipoprotein (a) in the population does not follow a standard bell shaped curve. More than two thirds of the population have low levels, while the other third has levels five times as high. This proportion has an interesting correlation with the observation that 36 percent of all deaths in the United States are due to coronary artery disease.

New studies have shown that the risk of having a heart attack is directly related to high plasma levels of lipoprotein (a). Many researchers are saying this test is more accurate in predicting the risk of a heart attack than any other blood test, including total cholesterol or its fractions, LDL and HDL.[8]

Attempts to reduce blood levels of lipoprotein (a) have not met with much success. Nicotinic acid, a form of vitamin B-3, is about the only material that has been partially effective in this regard. None of the cholesterol-lowering drugs available have yet been shown to lower levels of lipoprotein (a). This raises serious doubts about their effectiveness from yet another angle. It also raises a question of conflict of interest among lipid (fat) scientists who work for drug companies.

It is now possible to order tests for lipoprotein (a) in the blood. A few reference laboratories are doing the test, but few doctors have shown any interest in the test so far.

SUMMARY

The oxidation theory of the formation of fatty growths makes sense and should lead to the widespread use of effective preventive measures for coronary artery disease in the future. It helps explain many of the inconsistencies that have baffled scientists over the past 80 years. Because of the oxidation theory, medical scientists are now more receptive to studies reporting benefits from the intake of higher than usual levels of certain nutrients.

10

OTHER RISK FACTORS

The art of being wise is the art of knowing what to overlook.
William James

Commonly accepted risk factors for coronary artery disease include dietary consumption of saturated fats and cholesterol, as well as genetic tendencies, too little exercise, diabetes, obesity, high blood pressure, emotional stress, and smoking. However, experts tell us that in 40 percent of people who die of heart attacks, not one of these risk factors is present.

No one seems to be willing to stand up and shout at the experts, *"What the hell is going on here? You have spent hundreds of millions of dollars on research and you tell us this?"*

Our heart gurus may have the best of intentions, but they have come up with an inadequate list of risk factors. This is not discussed publicly. In my opinion, some of the standard risk factors appear to be valid. Others are only weakly associated with coronary artery disease.

SMOKING

Smoking is a well accepted risk factor. Evidence of damage from smoking comes from many sources. A smoker inhales not only nicotine, but 2,000 to 3,000 other combustion products present in cigarette smoke.

Cigarette smoke contains oxidized chemicals as well as free radicals. It is well accepted that chemical products in cigarette smoke can cause arteries to go into spasm. Epidemiological studies show an increased risk of heart attacks and cancers in smokers as well as inhalers of second hand smoke. If you smoke, quit. Everyone agrees with this advice except the tobacco industry that sells this addictive product, their representatives, politicians they have purchased, and hired lobbyists.

OBESITY

Obesity is another well accepted risk factor, but it probably isn't as important as people have been led to believe. The heart must work harder pumping blood through surplus fat. However, there are exceptions to the obesity connection.

Members of royal families in some South Pacific island paradises once spent their lives lying on the beach under palm trees and had underlings bring them food all day long. Kings and queens frequently weighted 300 pounds each. Diseases of physical degeneration were not seen until trading ships arrived with sweets and other refined carbohydrates. If obesity does play a role in heart attacks, it appears to be a minor one.

Everyone is aware of the poor experiences most people have in trying to loose excess weight. Actually, many factors related to obesity are poorly understood. Experiences in China demonstrate one exception to the *scientific* position that what we weigh is totally related to the balance between calories consumed and calories burned.

In China it is still unusual to see a truly obese person. Most Chinese tend to be skinny by our standards, yet a recent study found most Chinese consume 20 percent more calories than people in North America.

I have not heard nutrition experts try to explain this confirmed discrepancy. I do have a theory of my own. Most of the foods eaten in China are still fresh and unprocessed. By eating foods in the form to which we have adapted as a species we help maintain balance in the control mechanisms in the body that regulate everything. When we consume modern refined and processed foods we disrupt these control systems.

I have experienced this concept first hand during six trips to China. When I am in China I eat Chinese food three meals a day, every day (which is different from Americanized Chinese food available here). My Chinese friends joke about my large appetite. They pile surplus food onto my plate at the end of meals (for the *Honored Guest* every meal is a banquet). I eat much more food than I do at home, but usually loose about five pounds in a two to three week trip.

EXERCISE

Exercise is well accepted as being beneficial. More and more people are following exercise programs now than in the past. Exercise makes you feel good. In ancient times most humans had to work hard simply to survive. However, promoters have inflated any possible benefits exercise may have in preventing coronary artery disease.

I recently saw a graph showing the association between heart disease death rates and personal exercise levels. Higher death rates from coronary artery disease occurred on the extremes, among couch potatoes and obsessive over-exercisers. Between these extremes the death rate was a low flat line. Death rates did not decrease as levels of exercise increased as people who are *into* the exercise cult would expect. This demonstrates that aerobic exercise is no better for the heart than walking at a comfortable pace.

For many years promoters of exercise referred to a study among bus employees in London, England. Sedentary drivers had more heart attacks than conductors who walked up and down stairs and all over the bus all day.[1] This study was often quoted as demonstrating that exercise was protective.

More recently the study was discovered to have been flawed. Applicants for employment at the bus company were not assigned to their jobs in a random manner. Sedentary people applied for positions as drivers. Active individuals applied for jobs as conductors. This destroyed the validity of the study and it had to be thrown out.

Henry Soloman, a cardiologist at Cornell University Medical College in New York City, covered this subject in his book, *The Exercise Myth*. Soloman reviewed 2,200 medical articles studying the relationship between exercise and coronary artery disease. He found that exercise programs have not been found to slow the progression of the disease. Not only that, serious exercisers were 30 times more likely to die during their half hour of vigorous exercise than during any other 30 minute time period in the day.[2]

I recently saw two heart disease patients who had a history of collapsing during treadmill tests. Each had begun to experience chest pain and shortness of breath. Their cardiologists urged them to go just *one minute more* to reach some sort of level of performance the doctors felt was desirable. The men fell to the floor with cardiac arrest and pulmonary resuscitation. Even most non-medically trained people walking down an ordinary street intuitively sense it is not wise to over-stress a weakened heart.

THE PRITIKIN PROGRAM AND EXERCISE

The Pritikin Program manages heart patients successfully with diet and walking at a comfortable pace. Patients are encouraged to build up to where they walk six miles a day, if they can. They are discouraged from competitive situations, or bettering their times. The combination of diet and modest exercise seems to work just fine.

Medical Tribune once asked a leading exercise physician (guru) what he thought about the Pritikin Program. He said the exercise part of the Pritikin Program had to be the part that was beneficial, not the diet. This comment showed how totally unfamiliar he was with the program. He was not aware that many patients who entered the facility couldn't walk to the bathroom when they arrived. After they had been on the diet for a while they could begin walking bit by bit.

Therefore, modest amounts of exercise can be said to be beneficial. Too much or too little can be harmful. It is fine to exercise, but don't delude yourself that exercise is going to have much of a beneficial effect on coronary artery disease. The best evidence indicates that the progression of coronary artery disease is not slowed by exercise programs.

HIGH BLOOD PRESSURE

High blood pressure is another well accepted risk factor. The diastolic (lower) number of the pressure reading represents the pressure the heart must pump against at the beginning of each beat. An elevated diastolic (lower) number means the heart must work harder to circulate blood through the body. There is universal agreement that people with uncontrolled high blood pressure have a higher risk of a heart attack.

The problem with blaming high blood pressure as a risk factor is that its cause is usually unknown. Extensive testing finds a cause in only 5 to 10 percent of people.

The other patients are said to have *essential* hypertension, which is nothing more than a synonym of *God only knows* (abbreviated in medicine as GOK). Epidemiological studies of Cleave, and others, have shown that primitive lifestyle people did not have high blood pressure. This implicates the same types of diet and lifestyle changes we have been discussing.

Other studies have connected high blood pressure with deficiencies of specific minerals. Sometimes elevated blood pressures become normal without drugs when people take supplements of calcium, magnesium, or potassium. In my practice many patients have been able to slowly taper off their blood pressure pills when they switched to fresh food diets and took vitamin and mineral supplements.

DIABETES

Diabetics are highly prone to develop coronary artery disease. Again, the epidemiology of the development of diabetes is similar to that of hypertension and coronary artery disease. Successful primitive lifestyle people did not develop diabetes, though many of them must have carried genetic traits for the disease. Diabetes showed up only after modern foods containing refined carbohydrates entered the diet.

Diabetes is frequently easier to control when patients take supplements of the trace mineral chromium.[3] Chromium is incorporated into a material called the *glucose tolerance factor* that assists in the utilization of glucose (blood sugar). The trace mineral vanadium is also proving to be helpful in diabetic management. Another nutrient connection is in experimental diabetes in animals. In several species diabetes will occur when animals are placed on a diet that is deficient in vitamin B-6.

Therefore, a pattern emerges. The same changes in diets and lifestyles lead to the development of diabetes, high blood pressure and coronary artery disease. Genetic patterns determine what condition may develop in any one individual.

One small study demonstrated this relationship well. Two diabetics increased their intake of raw food and gradually were able to wean themselves off of insulin. Both had taken two injections of insulin daily for many years. As the percentage of raw food increased, the insulin need fell.

By the time the raw food portion of the diet had reached 80 percent, insulin requirements had decreased to zero. Because diabetics generally do better if they lose excess fat, researchers purposely kept the men's weights constant throughout the study to eliminate that factor.

These results are truly remarkable. Apparently no other researcher has ever tried to repeat this study. This is but one more demonstration of the dominance of the drug approach in medicine.[4]

INHERITED GENETIC FACTORS

A few years ago researchers discovered genetic markers for coronary artery disease. However, the trait must be a weak one because it can be manipulated by diet and lifestyle.

It is obvious that primitive lifestyle people carried genes for coronary artery disease, yet they remained free of the scourge. However, they followed some practices modern man does not. They consumed high levels of antioxidants and didn't eat oxidized foods. They also consumed higher dietary levels of vitamins and minerals that would allow slightly defective enzymes to function better (details of enzyme function are discussed in more detail in the next chapter).

STRESS

I believe emotional stress is not as closely related to coronary artery disease as most people believe. Western medicine follows a pattern. If a doctor can't figure out what is going on in a patient, the problem is blamed on stress. This is not good for patients, but it does keep the doctor on schedule in the office. One example of this oversimplification is that one hundred years ago the medical profession believed that angina pain was nothing more than a symptom of neurosis.

About 20 years ago we heard about *Type A Behavior* as a possible risk factor for heart disease. The theory said that the behavior of hard driving business executives was associated with an increased risk of heart attacks. Nobody seemed to care that a mechanism explaining how stress may cause fatty obstructions to grow in arteries has never been found. This is another example where a cause-effect relationship grew from noting more than a weak association.

By the early 1980s several studies had been published in which researchers attempted to verify the type A behavior hypothesis. All failed and the theory was quietly buried.

In many studies in humans arteriosclerosis has been blamed on stress after all other variables, including diet, were supposedly eliminated as risk factors. I have a problem with those studies because of the orientation of dietitians. The average run of the mill dietitian knows nothing of the work of Price and Cleave. Fat calories will get counted, but other more subtle changes in the diet will be missed if they are present.

Some animal studies support the hypothesis that stress may help cause arterial disease. Pigs kept in isolation developed more arteriosclerosis than pigs that live together. All were on the same diet. Similar results have been seen in monkeys whose territory was continually threatened. Rats have developed arteriosclerosis when they were crowded.[5]

These connections raise other questions, but they don't solve the problem. Study animals are in captivity and fed *rat chow* or similar man made heat-treated foods. These non-wild diets may lower resistance to disease enough that another variable such as stress may serve as the *last straw* on the camel's back (in the study group) that kicks them into a disease condition. I am not aware that animals living in the wild (on raw fresh food) have been found to develop arteriosclerosis.

EXCEPTIONS TO THE STRESS HYPOTHESIS

Doctors seem to have been happy to accept stress as a cause of heart attacks, but ignored exceptions to the theory. In Tokyo, on business days, people run around like frantic ants, walking a full 50 percent faster than my normal pace. The entire Japanese society demonstrates competitiveness that is said to lead to high stress levels and suicide rates. However, the death rate from coronary artery disease in Japan is only about 10 percent of the rate in the United States.

Another exception to the stress hypothesis occurred in England during World War II when death rates for coronary artery disease (and diabetes) fell by 50 percent. This occurred despite fears of a German invasion, losing the war, and German V-2 rockers blowing up city blocks without warning. It was a period of high anxiety and stress. However, as stress levels rose, death rates from heart attacks fell.

Many primitive lifestyle people have lived under conditions of stress. They had to contend with adverse weather changes, crop failures, lack of game, or attacks from other tribes, usually with brutal consequences, yet no coronary artery disease occurred. Cleave's opinion was that emotional stress will not produce organic disease in well nourished individuals.

One positive connection between emotional stress and coronary artery disease has been found. Poorly handled stress caused an increased loss of magnesium and other trace minerals in the urine. In a person whose magnesium status is marginal, this may be the last straw that initiates a catastrophic event.

REFINED SUGAR

John Yudkin was professor of nutrition at the University of London. Yudkin studied the relationship between refined sugar consumption and coronary artery disease for many years. He found the association was stronger than between cholesterol and fats and coronary artery disease.[6]

In his latter years Yudkin was frustrated in his attempts to inform colleagues and the public of his findings. Yudkin wrote that it became common for food processors to arrange to have entire conferences canceled when his name was listed as a speaker. Large food corporations use large amounts of refined sugar and the sugar industry *leaned* on them. Nutrition meetings usually are supported financially by food processors or their bulk suppliers.

When a chemist examines refined sugar he finds only sucrose. This sucrose identically resembles the sucrose found in the natural plant source (usually cane or beet). He then declares that refined sugar is no different than naturally occurring sugar.

There are other ways to demonstrate that the two forms of sugar are not the same, but the method is controversial and not accepted in conventional medicine. Electroacupuncture (according to Voll) testing of humans shows that about 70 percent of people have some sort of electromagnetic clash with refined sugar, whereas few show the same reaction to a piece of sugarcane. Apparently subtle electromagnetic properties of the sugar have been changed at the factory.

Perhaps this change is the result of heat, or formaldehyde and other chemicals used to clean out large cooking vats. Nobody knows. Therefore, to the chemist the two forms of sugar appear to be identical. To the theoretical physicist, they are different.

NUTRITIONAL DEFICIENCIES
Possible selective deficiencies of nutrients and other antioxidants are probably a major risk factor. These are discussed in Chapter 8.

CHLORINATED WATER
Chlorinated water is another possible problem. Chlorine is a catalyst for oxidation reactions. This means chlorine can help turn harmless fats into oxidized fats. Therefore, chlorine has no place in the body, even in tiny amounts.

Many people have had first hand experience with the toxicity of even small amounts of chlorine. Fresh water gold fish usually die if they are placed in chlorinated water that comes straight from the tap, though the concentration is only one part per million the same as in swimming pools. More recently, studies done with competitive swimmers using chlorinated pools in the U.S. have shown decreased lung capacity as the swimming season progressed. This occurred even as the swimmers trained harder and harder.

Consumption of chlorinated water has been linked to an extra 4,200 cases of bladder cancer, and 6,500 cases of rectal cancer a year, according to a new governmental study.[7] Many health conscious people avoid consuming chlorinated water by using bottled water, or boiling water before consumption.

European countries do very well with ozone purification of public drinking water. The ozone process is highly effective in preventing water-born infectious diseases. In contrast to chlorine, ozone dissipates spontaneously and leaves no residual in the water. It is unlikely Americans will change over to a non-chlorine method of purifying water because of the expense involved. Such efforts would also be fought by lobbyists representing manufacturers of chlorine who have a vested interest in maintaining the status quo.

OTHER CHEMICAL EXPOSURES
Since World War II a gigantic chemical industry has arisen. Chemical companies employ chemists who work in laboratories their entire lives doing nothing but making new chemicals. The company then tries to find commercial applications for these products, from making carpets and drugs to killing insects. At the present time there are over 70,000 different chemicals in production. In addition, we burn fossil fuels and other materials that release thousands of additional chemicals into the air.

At the present time it is impossible to avoid exposure to many of these products on a daily basis, even if a person is trying to do so. We are exposed to chemicals in the form of pesticide and herbicide residues in our foods. The majority of these compounds have never even been tested for safety.

The FDA allows about 2,500 food additives to be used in our foods and drugs (France allows only eight). These include known problem chemicals such as MSG and sulfites.

It is well accepted that sulfites can cause asthma attacks, and some of these attacks have been fatal. The FDA ordered restaurants to stop using sulfites on salads and vegetables a few years ago. At the same time the FDA has not forced the manufacturers of asthma inhalers to remove sulfites from the inhalers.

In order to save energy costs we have made our homes more air tight, reducing the number of air exchanges per hour. This has increased the level of chemical particles in the air, causing indoor air pollution. Many materials in the home out-gas toxic fumes, such as carpets and particle board.

Some European countries routinely check for chemical particles in the air of new office buildings and force them to be ventilated until the levels drop to acceptable concentrations. On some occasions occupancy has been delayed for up to six months. Until recently American employees were forced to move into chemically polluted new buildings. Those who complained the fumes made them ill were fired and had little chance to collect on workman's compensation claims.

There is a reason for mentioning chemical problems in a book on heart disease. Using sophisticated tests, chemical exposures have been shown to sometimes cause arterial spasm, and arterial spasm can cause angina or a heart attack. It is well accepted that cigarette smoke can cause spasm in small arteries in the hands and feet which can cause discoloration and even death of normal skin in a condition called Raynaud's Disease. Chemical exposures have also caused irregular heart rhythms in some people.

We all now have measurable levels of many chemicals in our body fat. This can be shown in fat biopsies analyzed in laboratories approved by the Environmental Protection Agency. A program of sauna detoxification has been shown to reduce the level of chemicals in the fat. As fat levels fall patients frequently improve.

The response of the chemical industry has been not only to stonewall the issue, but to try to suppress this information and the very approach itself. Some physicians working in the area have said that many defenders of the chemical industry have never have met a chemical they didn't like.

One physician, a medical director of a detox unit in California, became an effective witness in legal suits against chemical companies whose products had caused long term illnesses in people. As part of an industry backlash a licensure challenge was initiated against the physician. Rather than shell out $50,000 to $100,000 in legal fees in defense of his license, the doctor chose to retire and surrender his license. Fortunately, this occurred at a time when he had reached retirement age.

11

TRYING TO UNDERSTAND
CORONARY ARTERY DISEASE

Every new opinion, at its starting, is precisely a minority of one.
Thomas Carlyle

Enough data exist to construct a logical mechanism to explain how coronary artery disease develops. Once mechanisms are understood, logical preventive and treatment steps follow. I would like to develop this line of thinking briefly, then explore the hypothesis in more detail.

THE SHORT VERSION

Evidence exists that primitive lifestyle people remained free of heart attacks. Americans were also heart attack free up to about 100 years ago. The question now should be this: what can people do to prevent their genetic traits for coronary artery disease from giving them the disease? What are the common factors in diets and lifestyles that have been shown to prevent heart attacks?

Certainly, coronary artery disease involves a genetic component. If someone doesn't have the genes that promote coronary artery disease, it is probably impossible for such a person to get the disease, regardless how he or she may abuse the body. Winston Churchill is a good example of this. Churchill was an alcoholic, overweight, lived a sedentary life, chain smoked cigars, and lived a life of high stress. He may not have exercised because, as humorist Mark Russel has quipped, he was usually bombed before breakfast. However, Churchill outlived most of his cronies and died in his nineties. It is likely he did not have the genes for coronary artery disease.

Unfortunately, between one-third and one-half of us appear to carry genes for coronary artery disease, according to disease specific death rates. But the genetic trait did not lead to the full blown disease in the past. Our own ancestors carried these undesirable genes and remained heart attack free, at least until 1878.

Price, Cleave, McCarrison, and others discovered that the introduction of modern refined foods was followed by the development of diseases of physical degeneration. This change occurred regardless of the fat content of the diet of any other variables in lifestyle. This may be the most consistent pattern ever found in human biology.

Cleave discovered there was a lag period of about 20 to 30 years between the introduction of modern foods and the disease pattern shift. Price and Cleave were unable to carry their findings further because their discoveries were made before many other valuable pieces of the puzzle became available.

A comparison of the nutritional content of fresh foods to processed and refined foods explains much of what Price and Cleave observed. Modern supermarket foods commonly contain only 30 to 50 percent of the vitamins, minerals, trace minerals, and other antioxidants our ancestors consumed by eating fresh, natural foods. Primitive lifestyle people consumed levels of nutrients that allowed weak enzymes to function well enough to prevent coronary artery disease. When primitive lifestyle people made the switch to modern refined and processed foods, these weak enzymes could not function efficiently enough to prevent the onset of degenerative disease.

The new oxidation theory of atherosclerosis is consistent with this concept. In contrast to the primitive lifestyle diet, the modern diet contains oxidized foods as well as reduced levels of antioxidants. Examples are the elimination of vitamin E in white flour and the low average American intake of vitamin C of under 100 mg a day. This is far less than the 2,000 to 3,000 mg of vitamin C healthy people still consume in fresh food diets in the Tropics.

Therefore, the genetic tendency for coronary artery disease expresses itself when humans consume reduced levels of vitamins, minerals, and antioxidants that help to protect us from the disease. The concept is simple, yet it is not popular because the cholesterol theory, RDA concept, and establishment medicine's preoccupation with minutia have sent scientists off on unproductive tangents. Another stumbling block is the reluctance of nutritional scientist to admit that meaningful nutritional deficiencies are rife in America. The average American is overfed but undernourished at the same time.

THE LONG VERSION

Some knowledge of biochemistry is necessary to understand basic concepts in nutrition. Please don't fall asleep now. In medical school biochemistry was our most boring class. Students automatically fell asleep as soon as the slides came on and the lights went out during a lecture. Many doctor's brains still become mesmerized at the mere mention of the word *biochemistry*, as if they remain under the spell of a posthypnotic suggestion.

According to modern genetic theory, each enzyme within our cells is manufactured under the control of one gene. Over 10,000 intracellular enzymes have been identified to date. Each enzyme has the job of performing one tiny step in a specific chain reaction.

One enzyme may break a certain kind of chemical bond, another may stick some material onto a binding site of a molecule, another may remove something. The speed of these reactions is measured in pico seconds as various compounds pass down our internal chemical assembly lines at break neck speed.

If a gene is normal it will direct the production of a normal enzyme. If a gene is defective a substandard enzyme will be made. Enzyme activity is not an all-or-nothing situation. There is a gradation between efficient enzymes, to mediocre ones, to others that are so inefficient they are incompatible with life. In the most severe examples a pregnancy fails to begin. In other cases a woman's body somehow senses things aren't going normally and aborts the pregnancy spontaneously in the first few weeks after conception in what is commonly referred to as a miscarriage.

A normal biochemical process in the body is shown in Figure 1.

FIGURE 1

first compound ————————➤next compound
enzyme

The body does not manufacture complete enzymes. It makes what are called apoenzymes. Each apoenzyme must combine with its appropriate coenzyme to form a complete functioning enzyme. Most coenzymes are vitamins. Each enzyme also requires the presence of a specific trace mineral as a catalyst. A catalyst is a material that must be present for a reaction to take place, but is not consumed in the reaction.

So our drawing of the action of an enzyme now looks like this (Figure 2).

FIGURE 2

Trace mineral catalyst
substrate ————————➤next compound
apoenzyme + coenzyme

Many other factors determine efficiency of the action of an enzyme, in addition to the quality of the enzyme. Concentrations of the coenzyme (vitamin) must be within a normal range, not too much and not too little. Fortunately, the acceptable range is usually large. There must be adequate supplies of the raw materials (building blocks) the body needs to build an enzyme. Toxic metals such as lead, mercury, arsenic, cadmium, and aluminum, as well as fluoride and chlorine all can poison enzymes.

Many petrochemical products are toxic to humans for this reason. Pesticides and herbicides kill pests and plants because they poison enzymes that are critical to survival of those living organisms. These chemicals are also toxic to humans and animals because enzymes are shared throughout nature. Our bodies contain the same enzymes though they may not be as critical to our survival.

With this basic understanding of how enzymes work we can progress to a well accepted example of a genetic disease that is caused by a defective enzyme, methylmalonicaciduria. The name is long. Translated it simply means the chemical compound methylmalonic acid is found in high quantities in the urine of people with this genetic disease (Figure 3).

FIGURE 3

MMA ————➤Succinic acid
methylmalonyl CoA mutase

In this disease the enzyme is so inefficient it will only do about 1 percent of the work it should be able to do. Methylmalonic acid builds up in the blood and spills over into the urine. Because only small amounts of succinic acid are being made, levels of that compound will be low in the blood.

This is a serious condition. Children with this disease who are untreated develop mental retardation and die before the age of three. In most cases the condition is not suspected until one child has already died with the condition. With a subsequent pregnancy specialized biochemical testing can be done at birth to test for the defect (the mother's body can handle the biochemical abnormalities during the pregnancy).

Once diagnosed with laboratory tests, conventional treatment consists of daily injected doses of vitamin B-12, the coenzyme of the enzyme methylmalonyl CoA mutase. The amount of vitamin B-12 needed to correct the abnormal chemistry is individualized. The dose is determined by gradually giving more and more vitamin B-12 until blood levels of MMA come down.

Some children have had to take up to 500 times the RDA of vitamin B-12 daily by injection, a dose that must be continued throughout their entire lives. Some survivors are now in their 30s and perfectly healthy. For unknown reasons the treatment is not always successful.

This looks and smells like mega-vitamins to me, but orthodox physicians prefer to avoid that term. Semantics are very important to doctors, so the treatment is referred to as *enzyme induction* or some other synonym. There are 30 or 40 identified diseases that are similar that are referred to as *inborn errors of metabolism*. Each condition is treated with a very large dose of one specific vitamin.

Chemist Roger Williams described what he called the *law of gradients*. According to this concept a small number of people exist who might need 50 or more times the RDA of any one nutrient, a few more that might need 25 times the RDA, many who need the ancestral dietary level of three to four times the RDA, and a few lucky individuals who can get along well with far less than the RDA level.

The Food and Nutrition Board provides written material with the RDAs that explains that levels of nutrients listed should be adequate for 98 percent of healthy people. That is an interesting comment. By its own admission, RDA levels provide inadequate nutritional intake for the other 2 percent of us, and that adds up to about 5,000,000 Americans. There also seem to be a lot of us who can't really be called healthy because we live with some kind of long term ailment, especially as we get older.

NUTRITIONAL TREATMENT OF GENETIC DISORDERS

Most people, even physicians, believe that if a disease has a genetic basis, there is little that can be done to alter the situation. This may be true most of the time, but not all the time. It depends upon the strength of expression of the genetic trait. No one is claiming that nutritional manipulations can alter such strong genetic traits as sex, hair color, and size or shape of the nose. However, recent studies show that nutritional intervention can modify weaker genetic traits. Several examples of this concept are well documented.

Tipsy Mice?

Some mice carry a genetic trait for ataxia (dizziness). Mice that carry the trait stagger around as if they have been drinking highballs at a New Year's party. The defect shows up if their mothers eat what is normally considered to be an adequate diet for a mouse during pregnancy. However, if mother mice carrying the trait are fed high levels of the trace mineral manganese during a pregnancy, all offspring develop normal balance mechanisms.[1]

Prevention of Spina Bifida

Another example is our most common birth defect, spina bifida. Spina bifida results from a failure of normal development of the bones and nerves in the lower spine. The defect occurs when something interferes with the normal closure of a tube that forms our lower spine and nervous system. The defect occurs around 21 days after conception. Therefore, by the time a woman discovers she is pregnant it is too late.

In the 1970s British researchers discovered that women who were giving birth to babies with spina bifida had low blood levels of folic acid, one of the B vitamins. Their babies also had low to nonexistent levels of folic acid in samples of their cord blood. These deficiency levels were traced back to the mothers' dislike of leafy green vegetables and a failure to take vitamin pills containing folic acid.

Ordinarily, if a woman gives birth to a baby with spina bifida and has a second baby, the chance the new baby will have the defect is 5 percent. Researchers studied women who had already had a baby with spina bifida and wanted another child. The women took folic acid supplements daily, starting well before conception. The expected repeat rate of spina bifida fell by 75 to 90 percent in different studies.[2,3]

As frequently has happened in medicine, this discovery crossed the Atlantic Ocean to the United States with great difficulty (the NIH syndrome, Not Invented Here). Over the next 10 years, after a lot of infighting at the American Spina Bifida Association, studies were done in the U.S. that verified the British results.

Eventually the conservative Journal of the American Medical Association advised women to take multivitamins before and into a pregnancy to prevent spina bifida.[4] The Centers for Disease Control accepted the cause-effect relationship and advised that all women who are planning to become pregnant should take folic acid pills starting before the pregnancy.[5] More recently, the U.S. Public Health Service has advised that *all* women of reproductive age should be taking a folic acid pill every day.

There is no known risk to taking 400 to 800 mcg a day of folic acid as an oral supplement. If any physicians are fearful of advising women to take folic acid alone, they can recommend that it be given with some vitamin B-12. Better yet, they could recommend taking folic acid as part of a multivitamin-mineral combination.

NUTRIENT LOSSES
IN REFINED AND PROCESSED FOODS

As we have presented, the only consistent change that has led humans to develop coronary artery disease is the introduction of refined carbohydrates into the diet. The following tables demonstrate some of the nutrients lost when refined or processed foods are consumed:

TABLE 1
Nutrient Losses in White Flour Compared to Whole Wheat Flour

Fiber	87%
Protein	8
Thiamin (B-1)	0
Riboflavin (B-2)	0
Niacin (B-3)	0
Iron	0
Chromium	40-87
Manganese	85-91
Cobalt	56-88
Copper	67-85
Zinc	66-77
Molybdenum	43-48
Magnesium	83
Selenium	15
Silicon	99
Vitamin E	86
Pyridoxine	71-98
Pantothenic acid	64
Folic acid	46
Calcium	60
Biotin	70
Potassium	77

Thiamin, riboflavin, niacin, and iron are brought up to whole wheat levels by being added back through so-called enrichment.

Table adapted from: 1) Schroeder, H., *The Trace Elements and Man*, Devin Adair, 1973. 2) Ziegler, E. et. al., Amer Assoc of Cereal Chemists, 1971, in *Wheat Chemistry and Technology*. 3) *Nutritional Values of American Food*, USDA Handbook No. 456, Washington, D.C., Nov. 1975. 4) Schwara, Klaus, *Lancet* Feb. 26, 1977, p. 454-457. 5) Abrams, H. Leon, *Journal of Applied Nutrition* 1978, 30:41-55.

TABLE 2
Selected Nutrients in Canned Snap Beans (100 grams)

Calcium	37 mg	24 mg
Magnesium	25 mg	13 mg
Zinc	.024 mg	.020 mg
B-6	.074 mg	.030 mg
Folic Acid	36.5 mcg	18.2 mcg

Source: *USDA Composition of Foods Handbook*, U.S. Government Printing Office, 1984.

The standard American diet can be broken down as in Table 3:

TABLE 3

		vit/min content
Fats	40%	0
Sugar	18%	0
White flour	15%	20% of whole wheat
Commercially Canned or		50% of minerals lost
Frozen Veggies		80% of B-6 lost

Fats, sugar, and white flour products make up 73 percent of the average American diet and supply almost no vitamins or minerals. Even conventional nutritionists have expressed concern that the remaining 27 percent of the diet may not provide adequate levels of nutrients (RDA levels to them) to maintain health. Our disease pattern shifted gradually as these refined and processed foods were introduced into the diet.

When animals are placed on diets of refined and processed foods, they develop a long list of diseases of physical degeneration which increase in number and severity in successive generations. The relationships are so strong that specific nutrient deficiencies frequently can be shown to cause defects in specific parts of the body.

In spite of all of this, traditional nutritionists continue to tell us these changes in our diets can't possibly cause diseases of physical degeneration. They do so because academic nutrition departments teach that relatively low levels of nutrients are adequate, levels that prevent obvious deficiency diseases. By that standard a person is not considered to be malnourished in any one nutrient until his intake falls below 70 percent of the RDA level.

NIGHTMARES FOR NUTRITIONISTS

The new oxidative theory of the development of atherosclerosis and the disintegration of the cholesterol theory must be giving nutritionists nightmares. Higher than food levels of antioxidants are being shown to prevent coronary artery disease and extend life.

As the oxidative theory has become verified and accepted, nutritionists have failed to adjust. Have you seen any conventional source of nutritional information present a list of foods we should avoid because they contained oxidized cholesterol and other oxidized fats? Such action would offend the source of funding for nutritional research, biting the hand that has fed academic nutritionists for many years—the processed food industry.

How will nutritionists save face when they must finally abandon the cholesterol theory and move on to the more useful oxidative theory? How nutritionists and the American Heart Association handle this problem will be interesting to watch. Already there are indications they will simply say the oxidative theory has been hiding within the cholesterol theory all along, part of what they have been telling us for years. The last thing we can expect them to say will be that they have been painting themselves into a corner for 40 plus years and were wrong. That is a step most humans are unwilling to take.

SUMMARY

New discoveries make it possible to develop a plausible explanation for why we develop coronary artery disease. However, putting the puzzle together requires a multidisciplinary approach. Pieces of the puzzle have come from several fields such as epidemiology, biostatistics, nutritional sciences, food processing, medicine, laboratory sciences, and health politics.

I place most of the blame for our heart disease problem on changes the processed food industry has made in our food supply. Nobody is accusing the industry of intentionally plotting to oxidize fats and reduce nutrient levels of our foods. These disjointed changes occurred as part of the normal business activities of inducing us to eat more processed and refined foods so profit margins could be increased.

Nutrient losses caused by refining and processing foods were not discovered until at least 60 years after the fact. When the information did become available, the industry and its defenders (nutritionists) chose to believe the changes could not possibly be related to our changing disease pattern. Our taste buds by this time had become conditioned to foods that have been stripped of nutrients and doctored up with sugar, fat and salt. Instead of recommending a return to the consumption of foods in their fresh form, the usual quick fix was applied.

After all, people aren't dropping dead in the street from scurvy, beriberi, and pellagra, the old nutritional deficiency diseases. But we are dropping dead in the streets from heart attacks and magnesium deficiency induced arrhythmias and arterial spasms. Nutritionists and cardiologists have never connected these heart deaths with a life long pattern of sub-optimal nutrition caused by eating the average malnourishing American diet. They have defended the standard American diet as if it is somehow above criticism.

It will be most difficult for nutritionists to change their spots and recommend dietary steps and supplementation levels that will protect us from heart disease. I suggest that you not wait for them to see the light and come around. It is safe to proceed on your own because risks associated with these preventive steps are almost nonexistent.

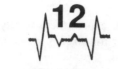

BIASES
AND POLITICS

Great spirits have always encountered violent opposition from mediocre minds.

Albert Einstein

Many positions presented in this book run contrary to standard thinking in medicine. These positions are backed by facts. When learning of these conflicts, many patients have asked why medicine seems to be doomed to advance so slowly.

As medicine has advanced through the past few centuries, poor judgement in the evaluation of new ideas has been the rule rather than the exception. The medical establishment almost routinely has rejected new ideas which were radically different from those accepted at the time.

Doctors hear about these mistakes of the past in courses in the history of medicine. For unknown reasons modern physicians believe these mistakes just can't happen today, as if basic human behavior patterns don't function within so-called modern *scientific* medicine.

Another obvious part of the problem is money. In the past the arguments about new ideas were strictly philosophical. Commercial interests seldom were involved. Now, multi-billion dollar multinational corporations have entered the picture and play dominant roles in maintaining what is good for them. In addition, physicians in several medical specialties have discovered they now have the opportunity to exploit their skills and *power* to become millionaires at young ages.

WIND UP SCIENTISTS

When new concepts or findings challenge vested positions, the response of the establishment is routine. Industries that have reduced the nutritional value of our food supply and polluted our environment have set up a series of organizations that claim to represent consumers but consistently defend the actions of industry. These outfits seem to keep batteries of *experts* in closets who are on call 24 hours a day to defuse public relations emergencies.

The experts are pulled from storage and wound up with little turn keys that stick out of their backs. During a warm up period they swagger back and forth from side to side making a mechanical whirring sound. Then they march out the door in unison to launch protective counterattacks.

Industry supported research is quoted on national television news programs. Press releases and faxes fly. Soon the issue becomes muddied beyond recognition. Typical of what happens to important issues that are covered in two minute news slots, within a day or two the conflict is no longer considered newsworthy. The little wind up scientist-dolls are stored away for future use, things go back to normal and the vested interests go on raping the system.

A perfect example of this modus operandi occurred in 1992. The Environmental Protection Agency was scheduled to release its findings on the risks of dioxin, a highly toxic chemical and a contaminant of *Agent Orange* of the Viet Nam era. Industry spokespeople preempted public presentation of the report by flooding the press with information that the study had found dioxin was not as dangerous as previously believed. Two weeks later the EPA reported that dioxin was in fact *more* dangerous than previously believed. By that time the public was totally confused on the issue.

FAMOUS HISTORICAL BIASES IN MEDICINE

Medical experts castigated William Harvey in 1628 when he claimed the heart pumped blood out to all parts of the body through tubes (arteries). Wanting to share his discovery with the world, Harvey traveled to the leading medical centers in Europe. The only reason he could even get his foot in the door of the European medical establishment was that he was personal physician to the King of England.

In his demonstrations he filled arteries of cadavers with colored water, then pumped the heart by squeezing it by hand. The colored water could be seen passing through arteries that had been exposed in various locations around the body. After observing what amounted to irrefutable proof of Harvey's claims about the circulation of the blood, professors of medical schools walked away and denied they had seen anything unusual.

Several decades later, when Harvey's findings finally were accepted, the circulation of the blood dominated medicine as a fad. Doctors believed all diseases were caused by problems with the circulation. Regardless of what was wrong with you, you were diagnosed has having circulation disorder type I, II, III, IV, or V. Each disorder was treated with blood letting plus one additional treatment, usually the administration of a toxic material. This approach dominated medicine for the next 200 years.

GEORGE WASHINGTON'S LAST BATTLE

George Washington's terminal illness exemplified medical treatment of the day. On December 12, 1799, George rode around his plantation in a freezing rain. The next day he developed a respiratory infection. In the early hours of December 14 Washington called for his plantation overseer, Albin Rawlings, who was proficient at blood letting. Fourteen ounces of blood were drawn.

At midmorning Washington's physician, Dr. James Craik, arrived and immediately called in two additional physicians as consultants. Before they arrived Craik
drew more blood. When the consultants arrived they drew more blood. They also
gave George a mercury compound to drink, as well as another medicine to induce
vomiting. Although the records are not exact, somewhere between five and nine
pints of blood were drawn from poor old George in about 12 hours. Washington
received the best care the medical establishment had to offer. He died around 11
p.m., about 20 hours after his medical treatment began.[1]

SIMMELWEISS AND BACTERIAL INFECTIONS

Ignas Simmelweiss was an Austrian obstetrician who played a prominent role
in the development of the next mega-fad, the germ theory. Simmelweiss concluded
that obstetricians were spreading a disease from the autopsy room to the delivery
room and this was causing large numbers of women to die.

This conclusion did not please Vienna's finest obstetricians. Having the finger
of guilt pointed at them was more than they could stand. Simmelweiss' theory was
unanimously rejected as hogwash. Arrogant physicians of the past have never
welcomed self criticism, and modern ones don't now.

The hospital had two delivery services. On the doctors' ward about 50 percent
of women having babies were dying of infections. Embarrassingly, across the hall,
where babies were delivered by midwives, the maternal death rate was less than 1
percent. Word go out about the high rate of death. Many women who were assigned
to deliver their babies on the doctors' ward chose to have their babies in the street
where they knew they had a much better chance of survival.

Physicians were baffled. Because of their training they knew they were
obviously smarter than the midwives and were practicing an advanced form of
scientific medicine. A major difference in the services was that midwives were not
allowed to do either autopsies or vaginal examinations before or during delivery, as
were physicians.

From today's perspective the problem was simple. Doctors were doing autopsies on women who died (part of the autopsy craze of the 1800s that documented the
absence of heart attacks) and gloves did not exist. After dipping their hands in the
pus of cadavers they simply wiped them off on their white (or off-colored?) lab
coats. Then they returned to the delivery area and performed vaginal exams on
women in labor and delivered babies. Hand washing was not practiced because
nobody saw any reason to do so (even to remove the stench). Bacteria and infectious
diseases were yet to be discovered. It is not reported if the doctors wore nose plugs
or not.

Simmelweiss suspected something was being transmitted from the autopsy area
to the labor area, though he had no idea what it might be. After several years of
developing his theory, he had a chance to put it to the test. His chief of service went
to London for three months and left him in charge. During that time Ignas forced
physicians in training to wash their hands in a chlorine solution before examining
women in labor or delivering babies.

Within days women stopped dying of infections. However, to maintain this progress, Simmelweiss had to watch his underlings 24 hours every day to enforce his order. Whenever he fell asleep, or was not present, doctors did not wash their hands and a few deaths would occur.

When his chief returned and found out what had been going on, Simmelweiss was fired on the spot. He continued to fight for his discovery, but was too far ahead of his time. The frustrations of his failed efforts drove him insane and he died 30 years later in a mental institution. Not long afterward bacteria were discovered and Simmelweiss became a hero. The all important mechanism had been found to explain the problem.

THE GERM THEORY

The germ theory replaced the circulation theory as the main fad in medicine. Soon doctors were trying to explain every disease on the basis of being an infection. For example, early in the 20th century, when Dutch researchers went to Indonesia to investigate an outbreak of beriberi (a vitamin B-1 deficiency disease), they were given orders to find and identify the bacterial cause of the disease.

We are still living in the era of the germ theory. The classic example is the treatment of a strep throat infection with a single antibiotic, penicillin. From this pattern an assumption developed in medicine that every disease should have a simple straight forward cause as well as a simple single treatment, similar to a strep infection. This is one reason why coronary artery disease and many other chronic diseases of physical degeneration have baffled researchers for years. They are complex diseases with multiple variables.

NUTRITIONAL BIASES

In the early phases of the development of academic nutrition scientists turned to the analytic approach. This refers to the process of describing foods in terms of the amounts of nutrients they contain. This was necessary to maintain control over the new science and the approach evolved into our current nutritional recommendations. Conventional sources say we should eat from the four food groups, or seven food groups, or the newer pyramid system, and get your Recommended Dietary Allowances of vitamins and minerals (RDAs). If you do this, all should be well with your nutritional status.

If you ask most nutritionists if there is a relationship between coronary artery disease and nutritional inadequacies they will say as a chorus, "NO! Go somewhere else. Everything is all right in the nutrition department. For God's sake don't look here. Why would you think anything so ridiculous. You must be a health food nut." In doing so nutritionists have overlooked useful clues from epidemiological approaches as well as animal research. I repeatedly found this pattern in reviewing material for this book.

When nutrition researchers studied primitive lifestyle people, they reported diets in simple terms such as percentages of the diet that were carbohydrate, fat, and protein. This was the result of believing in the preexisting dogma that processed foods are *just about the nutritional equivalent* of fresh foods. When they encountered healthy primitive lifestyle people who were eating all fresh foods, they didn't appreciate what they were observing.

If investigators had looked just one step further they would have stumbled onto something useful. No distinction was usually reported about whether carbohydrates were whole grain or refined. No mention was reported about how much of the diet was processed or cooked, fresh or raw. No comparisons were made of the total intake of every single little nutrient, right down to the most obscure trace mineral. Therefore, a body of cross comparison information on these questions does not exist.

VITAMIN C CONTROVERSIES

In 1974 a study was published in which vitamin C was mixed in a blender with food containing a known amount of vitamin B-12. The report claimed that vitamin C inactivated some of the B-12.[2] Other experts have quoted this report for years to discourage people from consuming greater than a recommended dietary allowance (RDA) level of vitamin C.

Two years later a duplication of the study was published in the leading nutrition journal, *The American Journal of Clinical Nutrition*. The author stated that in the previous study an inaccurate method of measuring B-12 had been used. Using the proper test he found that the addition of vitamin C had *no* effect on the content of B-12.[3]

Nutritionists who harbor strong biases against people taking nutritional supplements continue to refer to the first study and don't mention the second. In addition, there has never been any clinical evidence that taking vitamin C supplements creates problems related to vitamin B-12 in the human body, though some people have taken daily doses of 10,000 to 20,000 mg of vitamin C, and far more during viral infections.

DR. LINUS PAULING ON VITAMIN C

When Dr. Linus Pauling began to recommend large doses of vitamin C for the common cold and other conditions in the 1970s, the medical establishment united against him. Physicians accused Pauling, a chemist and winner of two individual Nobel Prizes, of going senile and venturing onto their turf.

Pauling is having the last laugh. When he was in his nineties he was still alert mentally and working on new discoveries in science. He lived to be 92. In later years he claimed to have increased his daily intake of vitamin C to about 20,000 mg.[4] The more he learned about vitamin C the more he took.

LINUS PAULING AND THE CHOLESTEROL THEORY

In 1975, having been thoroughly brainwashed by the establishment, I believed eggs, beef, cholesterol, and fat were dangerous foods. I attended a medical dinner meeting because I wanted to hear the after-dinner speaker. A friend had organized the meeting and made arrangements for Dr. Pauling to come and present his findings on vitamin C. I was asked to sit across from Dr. and Mrs. Pauling because my friend believed I was the only physician in the area who agreed with Pauling's views on vitamin C.

The waitress arrived and offered us two entrees, steak or fish. True to my biases at the time, I selected the fish dinner. Dr. Pauling chose the beef.

I watched Dr. Pauling cut into his juicy steak. This triggered my salivation response as if I was one of Pavlov's dogs. I asked why he chose to eat a food that was loaded with dangerous saturated fat. Pauling replied he believed that if we supply our bodies with all of the nutrients they need to function normally, our biochemistry will take care of cholesterol and fats and we won't have to worry about them.

I also asked him how it felt to be ahead of everyone else and controversial most of the time. He replied, "It is all right to be about 10 years ahead, not any more. If you get too far ahead, no one will catch up and give you Nobel Prizes."

To my knowledge Dr. Pauling has never *gone public* with a position that later proved to be wrong. That is why *real* scientists (physicians don't qualify to be called scientists) are reluctant to disagree with Pauling. They know he thoroughly researched the scientific literature on a subject before committing himself. When asked why physicians have not accepted the value of a higher than RDA intake of vitamin C, Dr. Pauling answers simply, "Ignorance of the facts."

A VITAMIN A OVERDOSE?

When my daughter was in the third grade the school nutritionist sent home a newsletter. The newsletter cautioned parents never to allow their children to consume more than one serving of a fortified cereal because that might expose them to a toxic dose of vitamin A (fortified foods have had RDA levels of certain nutrients added to them).

This sounded far fetched and sent me to my pharmacology text book. I copied pertinent pages and sent them to her. The lowest level of vitamin A poisoning ever documented was at a level about eight times the RDA for an adult, taken for many months. Even that case may have been a fluke because the next toxic level reported was in the range of 500,000 units a day for six months. The only deaths ever connected with an overdose of vitamin A were in Arctic explorers who ate large amounts of polar bear liver. But, in those cases, vitamin A intakes were not verified and autopsies were not done.

The nutritionist recanted her warning, then confided in me. She said her university teachers taught students to view RDA levels as amounts that should be reached in the diet but not exceeded. Higher than RDA levels were viewed as approaching toxic levels. The nutritionist said her school had never provided students with a list of verified overdose levels of nutrients, so she really knew nothing about the subject.

BIAS AT THE UNIVERSITY

In the 1970s a physician friend of mine told me about a nutrition class his daughter was taking at a state university in California. The instructor had passed out a one page list of books she warned students not to read. She wanted to protect their innocent minds from being exposed to what she called *nutritional nonsense*.

Included on the list were books by Nobel Prize winning chemist Dr. Linus Pauling, chemistry professor and nutrition pioneer Dr. Roger Williams, the chairman of McMasters University department of biochemistry, Dr. Russ Hume Hall, and many other highly qualified scientists.

PHYSICIAN BIASES

While I was practicing gynecology a general practitioner referred a lady to me because of vaginal bleeding. The patient had been told she was bleeding because she was taking 250 mg a day of vitamin C, a dose so far over the RDA it must be toxic.

This was obviously ludicrous, but it demonstrates how little most physicians know about nutrition and the strong biases they hold against taking supplements. In the United States a physician is probably the last person who should be consulted concerning nutritional matters. Most doctors would agree with this because medical schools offer almost no training in nutrition.

FOOD INDUSTRY BIASES

The processed food industry has a lot at stake in the issue of nutrition. Through research grants to major academic institutions the two have developed a close relationship. Departments of nutrition receive free visual aids which support the teaching of the four food groups and RDA concepts. They also receive large grants to study new products of interest to them, such as new uses for food additives. The result is that anyone who stands up and says eating processed foods can cause nutritional inadequacies and degenerative diseases is quickly labeled a quack and a charlatan.

Conventional nutrition continues to be taught with an emphasis on preventing obvious nutritional deficiencies. The bulk of interest is in the provision of adequate basic nutritional needs of people who are starving to death in famine areas of the world, or living in poverty situations in the United States. The idea that diseases of physical degeneration might be caused by sub-optimal intake of nutrients is regarded as a foreign concept. Much research supports this idea, but the food industry opposes it. If they were to accept this concept they would have to shut their doors or radically change their modus operandi.

BIASES IN MEDICINE

In the surgeon's dressing room of my hospital in California in 1976 I told some friends about a *miraculous* recovery. The wife of a medical school friend of mine nearly wasted away and died from a severe case of ulcerative colitis (ulcerative colitis can be described as a big, bad, crampy, bloody diarrhea that just won't quit).

My friend's wife was five feet eight inches tall. Her normal weight was 130 pounds, but she lost weight down to 80 pounds. She had to sit on the toilet for 12 hours a day every day because of diarrhea and cramps. She was taking cortisone by mouth and by enema. Nothing helped. She had even gone to see a shrink who confirmed that everything was all right in her head.

In this dismal condition her husband dragged her off to two ivory tower medical schools on the east coast for consultations from two of the country's most prestigious professors of gastroenterology (the study of diseases of the gut). Their advice was the same. It was time to remove her colon as a life saving procedure.

Rather than live with an *ostomy* and a collection bag for the feces, she refused surgery. My friend was forced to look for some alternative approach. By this time he was desperate and open to anything that sounded reasonable. He put his wife into a controversial hospital program in Chicago where she was fasted on pure water for several days, then fed one single food each meal as a challenge test. Ten offending foods were identified that triggered diarrhea, usually after just a few bites. She became well by avoiding those foods and has remained well since 1970.

When I finished the story an older urologist came over to me, put an arm around my shoulder, and gave me some fatherly advice. He said he knew everything I said was true because his sister-in-law also had recovered from ulcerative colitis through a food allergy approach. However, he warned me that if I continued to talk about such *miracle cures* and unorthodox approaches, I could get myself into a lot of trouble.

AN OPEN MINDED DOCTOR?

Not long afterward I began to try out some of the new approaches I was learning on relatives of my gynecology patients. I took an interest in hyperactive children and confirmed in my practice what Dr. Ben Finegold had discovered. Many children behaved better when they stopped eating what are commonly called *junk foods*. Such foods often contained chemical food additives (i.e., food colorings) and refined sugar.

I related my experiences to a pediatrician friend. Mike said he considered himself to be open minded, but he did not believe behavior changes could possibly be related to what a child was eating. Furthermore, he would not believe a cause-effect relationship was possible until he had seen 20 supportive double-blind studies in the journal of *Pediatrics*. By putting such impossible requirements in place Mike was safe in continuing to believe anything he wished.

EVEN MEDICAL LEADERS CAN STUMBLE

Dr. Arthur Coca found out about medical biases the hard way. Coca was one of the leaders in the field of allergy in the 1930s. He became editor of the major specialty journal in the field and a professor of allergy at a medical school. A diluting solution for allergy extracts, *Coca's Solution*, continues to bear his name to this day. Then he stumbled.

Coca, wrote a small paperback book instructing people how to self diagnose food allergies by detecting a rise in the speed of the pulse after eating a single food. The method works occasionally, but is not very accurate. At least the price is right.

Response from his allergy colleagues was not surprising. Coca was ostracized. Within two years he had been stripped of his professorship, was no longer editor of the allergy journal, and was no longer welcome at meetings of his peers.

I have presented these examples of non-heart related biases to give you an inside view of how medicine works. The medical establishment exerts extreme peer pressure on physicians to remain *conventional* and stay in line. After treatment approaches are firmly in place it is hard to dislodge them simply because they are proven to be worthless.

BIASES AGAINST SUPPLEMENTS

We have previously discussed the oxidation theory of the cause of atherosclerosis. New studies show taking beta-carotene may prevent many heart attack deaths. Another study showed taking some harmless vitamin and mineral supplements lowered the level of peroxides (oxidized fats) in the blood. Other studies showed women can prevent most cases of our number one birth defect, spina bifida, by taking pills of a safe B vitamin, folic acid, before and during early pregnancy. Why hasn't this information spread throughout the land and been made available to patients in every medical office?

The answer lies in a blind spot in medicine that results in a large bias against taking vitamin supplements. This bias takes many forms. Several years ago the late Carleton Fredricks described what happened on several occasions when he gave public lectures on nutrition during the 1940s. In his talks he stressed the value of eating fresh natural foods and taking vitamins and minerals. After each lecture he answered questions from the audience.

One night a lady asked him how she could get a wound to heal that showed no signs of wanting to heal. Fredricks always answered these questions in the most general of terms, being careful to never give direct advice to individuals. He quoted the literature and explained that several studies had shown taking some extra zinc could speed wound healing. This is perfectly true and defensible. However, as soon as the words were out of his mouth, several policemen came from backstage, arrested him and hauled him off to jail. Unknown parties had arranged for him to be arrested and charged with practicing medicine without a license.

THE VITAMIN B BUST

On May 6, 1992, twelve unarmed Food and Drug Administration agents and ten armed King county Sheriff's Department officers wearing bulletproof vests broke down the front door of a medical office in Kent, Washington, with a sledge hammer. The clinic was scheduled to unlock its doors in another ten minutes. The law enforcement agents stormed in, pointed loaded weapons at receptionists, and told them to keep their hands in view. When Dr. Jonathan Wright arrived a few minutes later he found a chaotic scene. He was also prevented from entering his office.

The FDA agents had obtained a search warrant from a Federal judge on grounds that illegal drugs were being manufactured on the premises. The FDA agents had requested assistance from the sheriff's office and the sheriff's deputies had come prepared for a major bust of street drugs. For 14 hours agents searched every inch of the office, finally removing enough boxes of records, supplements, and equipment to fill a moving truck.

After FDA officials refused to comment on the raid for several days, reporters pressured them into revealing what they had found. All they could mention was they had found some preservative-free injectable B vitamins from Germany and three galvanic skin sensing machines used for allergy testing. The machines were considered to be illegal because they had not gone through the FDA approval process, though they had been sold openly in the United States for 10 years.

Why did the FDA agents use Gestapo tactics and behave as if they were raiding a cocaine ring? Some people associated the raid with a lawsuit Dr. Wright had filed against the FDA. In 1991 Wright sued for recovery of some uncontaminated tryptophan (an amino acid) which had been seized by the FDA. One month later FDA agents started to go through Wright's garbage, looking for anything incriminating they could find.

Others suspected a more sinister plot was involved to try to wipe out alternative/holistic physicians and health food stores. Such an action would allow the drug industry to maintain its domination of our medical system. In any event, the raid was a highly unusual action. In a public statement, Dr. David Kessler, chief of the FDA in Washington, D.C., defended the actions of his agents, saying they were justified in everything they had done.

NO VITAMIN C ALLOWED

A doctor friend of mine left general practice to take a residency training program in radiation oncology, the treatment of cancers with radiation therapy. After reading some medical articles he became curious about the possibility of reducing side effects from X ray treatment with vitamin C.

On rounds one day he raised the subject. His professor ignored him, not even acknowledging the question. A week later he brought up the subject again. This time the professor did respond. He told him to get his mind off of vitamin C. In addition, if he ever mentioned vitamin C again, he would be expelled from his training program.

Dr. D., a gynecologist friend of mine, discovered many years ago that taking 750 mg of vitamin C daily prevented his gums from bleeding when he brushed his teeth. Any time he forgot to take his vitamin C his gums would bleed. In 1978 he had a heart attack and was taken to Stanford University Medical Center where he had cabbage surgery.

When he regained his senses he asked his surgeon to write an order allowing him to take his usual vitamin C dose. Dr. D. knew extra vitamin C also could speed the healing process. One of the leading cabbage surgeons in the country told him, "We are running a surgical service here. We don't deal with nutrition." Dr. D. was forced to take his vitamin C on the sly.

BIASES AT THE FDA

On two occasions during the past 20 years the FDA has tried to restrict the availability of vitamins and minerals in doses greater than one RDA. Their efforts failed because of letter writing campaigns from the public. In 1992 three bills were introduced in Congress. All three died at the end of the congressional session, but similar bills are expected to be reintroduced.

1. No More Herbs?

The first bill would have prohibited the sale of all herbs in the United States. The reason offered for this unusual action was that possibly four of five herbs have toxic side effects and can be poisonous if used improperly. Problems can also arise if herbal remedies are not extracted properly. This difficulty could easily be resolved by some sort of inspection for quality. The FDA seems to forget the Chinese have used over 2,000 herbs safely (and effectively) for centuries. Native Americans and many other people from around the world have routinely used herbs with safety.

The drug industry has a lot to gain from this bill. Eighty-five percent of all people in the world treat themselves with inexpensive herbs instead of more expensive Western drugs. The pharmaceutical industry doesn't want that trend to spread to the United States. The drug industry currently has gross revenues of over $130 billion a year and has the highest rate of return on investment of any industry. That creates a lot of money and incentive to throw their power around in Washington lobbying congressmen and influencing people at the FDA.

2. No More Amino Acids?

A second bill would have prohibited the sale of all amino acids. Amino acids are the small building blocks of proteins. The basis of this proposed legislation is a problem encountered in users of the amino acid tryptophan. In 1989 over 1,500 tryptophan users became ill and at least 38 died.

The FDA soon traced the problem to consumption of tryptophan. It removed all supplies from the market which, everyone agrees, was a proper action. A short while later the problem was found to be related to a batch of tryptophan from Japan that was contaminated with a toxic chemical from a renovated chemical tank.

Tryptophan is an essential amino acid that had been on the market for many years with no problems. Even though it has been described in medical journal articles and psychiatric textbooks as being useful in the treatment of depression and sleep disorders, the FDA continues to claim tryptophan serves no useful purpose. Even after the FDA found the contamination problem, its spokespeople have continued to refer to the incident as the tryptophan problem, instead of the *contaminated* tryptophan problem. Tryptophan supplements continue to be banned from the market.

Recently, the FDA offered an explanation for this action. Up to 5 percent of people who were poisoned took tryptophan that did not come form the one batch in question. Some cases occurred prior to the epidemic of 1989-90 and some similar cases have been linked to a compound related to tryptophan.[5]

Proponents of the use of tryptophan have responded that the other cases also were clustered in a short time period which suggests they were caused by a previously contaminated single batch. This may be a reason for careful monitoring for impurities, as would be done if an FDA approved drug was involved. This is how the FDA handled the Tylenol poisonings in the early 1980s, instead of banning the product indefinitely.

Another quirk of the FDA was revealed by its actions concerning tryptophan. While tryptophan oral supplements were banned, no restriction was placed on the use of commercially manufactured tryptophan in infant formulas and intravenous feeding solutions. Some of these batches of tryptophan apparently were coming from the same supplier that was responsible for the chemically contaminated material. This once again demonstrates biases the FDA holds that lead them to help the pharmaceutical industry and demolish its competitors.

3. Restrictions on the Sale of Vitamins and Minerals?

The third bill would have restricted over-the-counter sales of vitamins and minerals. Only multivitamins and minerals containing one RDA or less of any compound would be allowed to be sold to the general public. Higher doses would require a doctor's prescription. Keep in mind that only 15 percent of physicians take vitamins themselves, and most openly scoff at the idea. Under such a regulation, if an elderly man wished to take 500 mg of vitamin C daily to try to live six years longer, he would need to go to his doctor, ask for a prescription, and be laughed at.

Together these bills appeared to serve but one purpose. The health food industry in the United States would be crippled if bills similar to these were to pass. If enacted into law Americans would become more dependent on drugs made and sold by the FDA's bedfellow, the pharmaceutical industry.

It is ironic this is happening at the same time the oxidation theory of atherosclerosis is becoming so widely accepted. Protection of arteries from oxidative damage requires that people take several multiples of the RDA of several nutrients. You might not be able to get these antioxidants without a prescription in the future if future versions of these bills pass.

CONTROL IS THE WORD

Part of the bias behind these bills comes from another hidden agenda that is unrelated to the large drug companies. Medicine likes to manage the field of health. Many doctors feel uncomfortable with patients who question medical recommendations and follow diets and other health practices designed to take charge of their own health.

Some patients have told me that when these issues have arisen they have received registered letters from their doctors telling them to get new doctors. This is a legal way for a doctor to break off the legal doctor-patient relationship. Such patients are viewed as being out in left field, or some sort of health nut kook. To some doctors being exposed to these concepts is similar to hearing the sound of fingernails scratching down a blackboard.

The key word here is *control*. In 1977 the State of California established a licensing board for acupuncture. Several physician friends of mine served on this new board and conducted its licensing examinations. Soon a representative of the California Medical Association showed up at one of their board meetings.

He said the California Medical Association wanted the acupuncture board to place itself under its jurisdiction. Board members asked if the CMA had any interest in acupuncture, or possibly wanted physicians to learn acupuncture. The reply was that the CMA knew nothing about the ancient practice and had no interest in learning about it. It simply wanted to *control* all aspects of health care in the state.[6]

MEDIA BIAS

Arline and Harold Brecher wrote about control of the media in their book, *Forty Something Forever*. The Brechers are journalists who began to write on health issues many years ago. Editors rejected many of their articles because they ran contrary to the positions of powerful vested interests or organizations.

When they submitted articles to a newspaper about nutrient deficient foods, editors would not publish them because of fears of offending supermarket advertisers. Editors required articles about cancer to be screened and approved by the American Cancer Society. Articles on heart disease had to be approved by the American Heart Association.

The Brechers described a situation where Hollywood screen writers were forced to rewrite scripts of a new dramatic medical television series. In the original script the central character and hero was going to be a doctor who used alternative medicine methods. This was found to be unacceptable to the powers that be. The script was rewritten to make the doctor more conventional.[7]

Russell L. Smith, Ph.D., has described efforts he has made to publicize information showing the cholesterol theory is a scam. He contacted a variety of magazines offering to write a series of articles. All refused to publish stories, articles, or letters to the editor.

One popular women's magazine stated its position very clearly in a rejection letter. An editor wrote that the magazine did not publish information about heart disease that ran contrary to public positions of the American Heart Association.[8]

MEDICAL BIASES AND POLITICS

Drug companies control what gets published in medical journals through their advertising dollars. An interesting situation surfaced several years ago when a medical journal published a double-blind study showing an herb had beneficial effects in the condition being studied.

One of the journal's drug company advertisers contacted editors. The drug company threatened to *never* advertise in the journal again if they *ever* published a similar article. The editors caved in to the economic pressure. The difference was that in this particular case the story leaked out and became public.

Most medical journals now contain about one-third printed material and two-thirds slick advertisements for drugs. According to the Wall Street Journal, drug companies spent over $330,000,000 on advertising directed at doctors in 1990. You can rest assured major medical journals that rely on drug industry money are not going to publish articles that demonstrate benefits from competing treatments such as diets, herbs, acupuncture, chelation, vitamins, minerals, amino acids, or other *complimentary* approaches.

CONTROVERSIAL TREATMENTS AREN'T CROSS INDEXED IN MEDICAL LIBRARY COMPUTER BANKS

Most physicians are not aware that only a small number of medical journals are cross indexed into medical computer banks. About 3,000 medical journals are published each month, and only about 10 percent of these make it into the indexes.

Conservative editorial boards keep articles on controversial topics out of the major medical journals. The articles must be published in journals that are not cross-indexed in computer banks. Therefore, they will not show up when orthodox physicians ask medical librarians to conduct computer searches, or in CD-ROM services such as *Medline*.

Dr. Richard Casdorph encountered this editorial bias several years ago. Casdorph is an assistant professor of medicine and cardiologist at the University of California School of Medicine, Irvine, California. By chance, Casdorph ran into some old articles on chelation therapy. He decided to evaluate chelation therapy himself with modern evaluation methods which were not available when the older studies were done. At the time he was not aware of the political black cloud establishment medicine has placed over chelation therapy.

In one study Casdorph measured blood flow through the brain with radioisotopes before and after 30 chelation treatments. Blood flow increased in 85 percent of the patients. In another, he measured ejection fractions (pumping efficiency) of the left ventricle of the heart before and after 20 chelation treatments. Ejection fractions improved in almost all patients.

In a third study he reported how chelation saved the legs of four patients who were scheduled for amputation because of gangrene. Pictures taken before treatment showed feet and toes with black areas of dead tissue. Photographs taken after treatment showed the gangrene had healed and the patients still were walking on their own legs.

Casdorph submitted the heart study to the *New England Journal of Medicine*, expecting almost routine acceptance. He was shocked when a rejection notice came back by return mail. He mailed the article to several other major journals and all responded with a rejection letter.

He called friends on editorial boards of the journals to inquire about what was going on. The reply was that chelation was known to be a dead issue. It had been found to be ineffective many years before and, therefore, was an inappropriate therapy. Casdorph eventually published his articles in the Journal of Holistic Medicine. He joined the group of chelating physicians and later served as its president.

PRESSURES TO REMAIN ORTHODOX

Doctors function under a tremendous amount of peer pressure. Medical professors try to turn medical students into clones of themselves. The profession then expects the little clones to follow the *American Medical Association party line* forever. If a physician decides to become a maverick he opens the door to trouble.

The late Dr. Robert Mendelsohn wrote about this problem in his book, *Confessions of a Medical Heretic*. Mendelsohn started out as a conventional doctor,

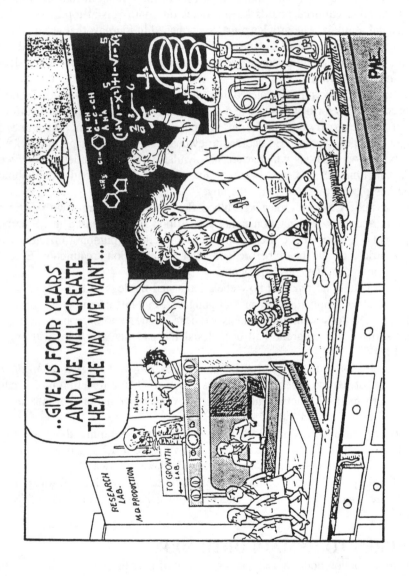

as we all must. He worked his way up in academia to where he was a professor of pediatrics at the University of Illinois Medical School. He also sat on the Illinois State medical licensing board. Those are good, solid, mainstream credentials. After years of orthodox activities he decided to spill the beans on medicine.

Mendelsohn referred to medicine as a religion, calling it the *Church of Modern Medicine*. In this church medical school professor are the high priests. They decide what dogma will be canonized. Medicine builds walls around the dogma and demands that doctors confine their diagnostic and treatment methods to those currently approved by the system. If a doctor ventures one inch outside the walls, he is eligible to be burned at the stake. For example, if a doctor does conventional general practice 99 percent of the time and some alternative technique 1 percent of the time, that is enough to be called a quack.

Medical mavericks are being harassed with increasing frequency. The public is becoming disenchanted with the direction medicine is taking (more costly and dangerous diagnostic procedures and treatments), and more physicians are defecting from the dogma. Many defectors are paying a high price simply for providing their patients with a high quality of medical care that is frequently more effective, safer, and cheaper. A good example is the ordeal of Dr. Warren Levin of New York City.

THE CASE OF DR. WARREN LEVIN

The New York State Attorney General's office charged Dr. Warren Levin with fraud for the way he practiced medicine in his office. This in itself was a highly unusual step.

The state claimed Levin was using diagnostic and treatment procedures he knew were not valid. Therefore, these actions represented not malpractice, nor unethical practice, but fraud. This action did not originate from a malpractice action or a patient complaint. The complaint came from one individual, a non-patient, whose identity the state refused to reveal. The trial was conducted in segments over a three year period. Levin had to hire attorneys for his defense, and legal fees have sent him into bankruptcy.

One of the issues pertained to Dr. Levin's use of intravenous chelation therapy as a treatment for arterial disease. Several university professors testified in defense of Dr. Levin, presenting research that showed beneficial responses in patients treated with chelation therapy.

To counter this testimony the state called a physician with impressive credentials as its expert witness on chelation therapy. The expert had written many journal articles (none about chelation) and held an academic position at a highly regarded medical school. Dr. Levin's attorney extracted surprising information from this witness on cross examination.

The expert had not bothered to ask his medical librarian to pull recent articles on chelation therapy so he could review the subject. He had not read a copy of the trial transcript pertaining to information favorable to chelation therapy that had already been presented by other experts. He had never talked with a patient who had received chelation therapy. He had never given a chelation treatment. He had never

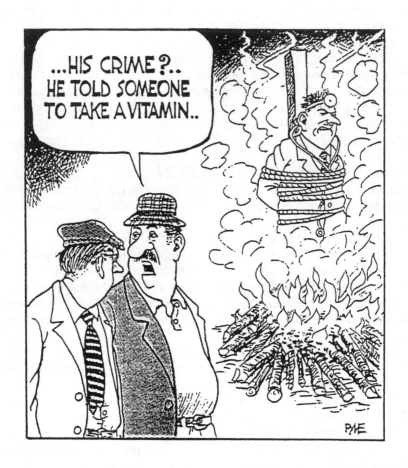

talked with any physician who had any direct experience with chelation therapy. It soon became apparent the expert witness had no direct knowledge about chelation therapy at all.[9]

After the defense had shown that the state's expert witnesses were not qualified to judge how he practiced, the state ruled against Levin. The *jury* was composed of three conventional physicians.

Many more examples of this sort of harassment of innocent physicians are described in James P. Carter's book, *Racketeering in Medicine*. Also described are the efforts of a collection of conspiratorial vested interests who are intent on destroying any practices and anyone that does not support the medical/pharmaceutical/industrial/complex.

SOMETHING ROTTEN IN DENMARK

An article on chelation therapy published in 1991 had a bad aroma. The conclusion of the article was that chelation therapy didn't work. The investigators were a group of Danish vascular surgeons, not exactly an unbiased group when it comes to evaluating a competing treatment that might cut into physicians' income.

These surgeons claim to have conducted a double-blind controlled study using EDTA chelation therapy.[10] Patients all had intermittent claudication which is caused by obstructed arteries in the legs. Victims are able to walk a certain short distance, then must rest because of pains in their legs.

Because results reported were so different form all other published studies about chelation, another Danish physician tried to learn more details of the study. He first asked the surgeon-authors if he could see raw data from the study but was denied access. He then tracked down the interviewed several patients who had participated in the study.

From various statements given by the patients, it looks like the patients were not kept in two treatment groups. Even the two articles published on the study state the *blind* nature of the study was broken early in the study. Apparently chelation and saline drops were alternated in many patients. Therefore, there were no separate groups receiving different treatment.

The investigators did some other odd things. Patients were requested to chew iron tablets while their drips were running. If you want to destroy the effect of chelation therapy this is probably the best way to do so. This was a highly unusual action.

The report also concluded records may have been falsified. One patient said she told her doctor she was getting better, but saw him write a note in the chart saying she had not improved.

The way the study was reported also arouses suspicion about the honesty of the investigators. Of 153 patients in the total study, 70 percent were smokers. The first published study reported on only 30 patients, 29 of who were smokers. The odds of this distribution occurring by chance alone is 1 in over 14,000 (smoking also reduces the odds that chelation therapy might help).

The published articles reported that *all* patients averaged a 51 percent improvement in maximal walking distance after the first 10 treatments. There was "no difference between the EDTA and saline groups."

This is a highly unusual finding and is what would be expected if patients' treatments were crossed over, back and forth between EDTA drips and saline drips, as mentioned above. The authors attributed this improvement to the widely seen phenomena of *"spontaneous recovery."*

I have never seen a single spontaneous recovery in *any* patient with this condition, nor have I ever heard of a single case since I entered medical school 35 years ago. Such a dramatic result is never seen when doctors give patients the drug Trental, which is approved for this condition by the FDA.

It is disappointing that the editors of the two medical journals that published articles from this study accepted them without questioning this highly irregular finding.[11] Unfortunately, this is simply *the way things go*. Medical journal editorial boards must be so eager to receive a report blasting a treatment that is scorned they will abandon their normal levels of evaluation in the scrutiny of articles submitted. This is not the first time this has occurred.

The end result is that this article has been used to hurt chelation therapy. Opponents of chelation therapy claim that this is the only double-blind study of chelatin therapy that has been published (even if it was an inaccurate study). They are not aware another double-blind study has been published that showed that chelatin did work. Unfortunately, because the results supported chelatin therapy, it was published in an obscure journal.

WHO DETERMINES MEDICAL POLICIES?

Very few people may be responsible for a wide reaching policy. At a medical organization interested in heart disease a small committee may be appointed to study chelation and present its findings. In dealing with an unaccepted treatment such as chelation, it is likely all the committee does is meet and issue a quick statement, without bothering to read the medical literature. The policy of the organization then becomes set in stone.

When other physicians ask questions about the therapy, the organization mails them a pamphlet, or provides this information over the phone. Most doctors will automatically follow these conclusions like sheep. Physicians say they are too busy to go to the library and pull out articles that might change their minds, the same as most have never read the weak studies used to support the cholesterol theory, or the articles showing the ordinary angiogram is unreliable.

Medicine functions like other human institutions. It continues to show an inability to fairly evaluate valid new concepts. Many times it adopts invalid concepts, puffs them up into fads and defends them to the death, at the same time stomping out any competing ideas. Good examples of this type of behavior are the cholesterol theory and treatment of coronary artery disease with surgical procedures.

Therefore, you need to become better informed and take charge of your own health. Practice protective measures that have been proven through the ages to help prevent and even reverse coronary artery disease, even if your doctor may not understand what you are doing or understand what you are talking about.

ILLUSIONS

Western medicine creates an illusion that it is based on hard science and great knowledge. If you ever have the opportunity take a walk through the halls of a large university medical center, you will get lost in the multitude of hallways and departments as you pass serious looking people wearing white lab coats. The very walls seem to exude a feeling of great knowledge and an honest search for the truth. By God, if the secrets of the body are going to be unlocked, it is going to happen here!

Most people are unaware that so called "medical science" is based only on what can be seen and measured, and this probably represents only a small fraction of what is really going on. Western medicine looks at the body as if it is a sack of skin filled with tissues in which thousands of complicated biochemical processes keep humming along. The processes are influenced by hereditary patterns, nutrients, toxins, light, heat, and other environmental factors. No effort is made to explain how this complicated system works, how it may be coordinated. This has not stopped medicine from creating the illusion that it is a scientific discipline, based on concepts that are understood and proven to be valid.

This question of how things are *proven* in science led to a conference on the subject several years ago. Albert Einstein was invited to give his views in a speech. Organizers of the meeting thought the question was a simple one. Einstein did not. He respectfully declined to attend because he *"thought the question was too profound."*

A DOUBLE STANDARD

A double standard is at work in what becomes accepted as medical dogma and what does not. Most of the treatments currently used in medicine have never been subjected to the same scrutiny that would be required if they had been discovered now. I am not saying many of these treatments are ineffective, only that most don't meet the criterion of having been *adequately tested* by modern day standards.

Yet, unpopular treatments are required to go through extensive testing before they may or may not be accepted. In some cases these treatments may have been in use successfully for thousands of years in other cultures. In almost all cases the tests are never conducted because people who control the sources of research funding make it impossible for studies to ever be conducted.

TRADITIONAL CHINESE MEDICINE

In contrast, traditional Chinese medicine views the body as being primarily an energy system. This subtle energy system is either in harmony or disharmony with the environment. The energy system regulates and coordinates all bodily functions and processes. When the system is out of balance we become ill. It is the energy system that controls our biochemistry and our fate. It is this body energy that ceases to function when we die.

Western medicine has strong biases against studying anything to do with such an energy system. The problem goes back almost 100 years ago to the time of black boxes and large amounts of quackery. Charlatans roamed the United States traveling from town to town promoting the healing powers of electronic devices, black boxes with flashing lights and dials.

Commonly, two wires led from such instruments to brass cylinders which were held in the hands of sick people who were seeking cures. As the operator turned up a dial, victims received an electric shock, then were told their ailments had been treated successfully. Money changed hands. Ever since that time medicine has taken a dim view of energy treatments and the entire subject of body energy.

In more modern times research funds have been unavailable to study subtle energy relationships in the body. A few years ago a study was planned to see if microwave radiation might be causing Army helicopter pilots to father an excess number of children with birth defects. During their training the pilots had to fly repeatedly directly over high output microwave transmitters used for communications. The Department of Defense blocked funding and killed the study without comment.[12]

More recently the Federal Food and Drug Administration has been confiscating harmless galvanic skin measuring instruments from physicians' offices. These pieces of equipment have been used in a system of German Electro-Acupuncture I have observed to be beneficial, many times when all other treatments have failed.

WE DON'T REALLY KNOW MUCH

Western medicine has made many great discoveries. However, it is said that each new discovery uncovers 10 more things we don't know. We may discover the chemical composition of a gene, but have no idea why or how it functions. We know what enzymes are, but have no idea how or why they function.

We can observe healing after surgery, but can't explain why it occurs. The surgeon may sew tissue edges together. The body mysteriously does the healing. We don't know why we make growth hormone for several years, then stop before we are 10 feet tall.

When we discuss higher functions, we know even less. We have no idea how or why we learn. We don't know why we forget. We have no idea how our memory works, or how we think.

We use electricity and explain it as a flow of electrons, but don't have any idea what it really is. We can't answer the simple question, "What is life?" Can anybody explain the mystery of love? The list is long.

When I hear or read smug comments from so-called medical experts, I think about Dr. Robert Mendelsohn who became a self proclaimed *medical heretic*. Mendelsohn said this would never have happened to him if he had not flunked his course in arrogance in medical school.

My advice is to keep an open mind and be willing to look into complicated issues on your own. Don't rely on the opinion of committees of experts. Do a lot of reading. As you have seen, medicine's approach to the prevention and treatment of heart disease involves layers of fraud and deception, and leads to a lot of suffering and needless expense. There are better ways.

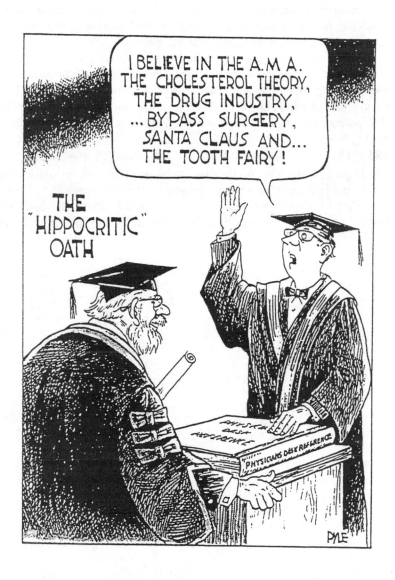

ORGANIZED BIAS

In recent years a new twist has been added to biases that function in medicine. The pressures that work against the acceptance of new ideas have become organized and coordinated. Industry funded vested interests control what is published, what appears in the media, and in medical journals. Useful, cheaper, alternative medicine approaches that may have been used successfully for hundreds or thousands of years, are being attacked in meetings directed at the public.

Cosponsors of these meetings are the National Council Against Health Fraud, the American Medical Association, the American Pharmaceutical Association, and the Food and Drug Administration. This strange collection of bedfellows has joined together to warn the public about the dangers of vitamins, minerals, herbs, acupuncture, chiropractic, chelation therapy, and homeopathy.

SUMMARY

The history of medicine is rife with biases and there are no signs things have changed. In the past differences were philosophical and between individuals. Now, vested interests have created organizations to attack treatments and individual practitioners who are perceived as threatening the status quo, and this translates into protecting profits.

13

REASONABLE ACTIONS

The doctor of the future will give no medicine, but will interest his patient in the care of the human frame, in diet, and in the cause and prevention of disease.

Thomas Edison

I have attacked myths about heart disease that cost Americans billions of dollars per year in unnecessary surgical procedures, as well as untold suffering. The list of abuses can start with the widespread use of inaccurate angiograms which are used to plan surgical procedures. People are conditioned to expect to live longer if they have cabbage surgery, but survival rates are not improved with surgery. The system encourages doctors who are learning to do balloon angioplasties to practice on people who don't need *any* surgical procedure. Long term survival after balloon angioplasty has never been studied. The cholesterol theory is an empty shell. These approaches to our number one killer disease represent a fraud against the people more often than not.

There is a brighter side. Studies of primitive lifestyle people show their diets and lifestyles protected them from coronary artery disease. Even American pioneers of 100 years ago who carried the genetic trait for excessively high blood cholesterols lived to ripe old ages. One obvious pattern we should follow is to try to copy what our ancestors were doing as much as possible. They must have been doing a lot of things right.

Recent discoveries in the area of the oxidation theory of coronary artery disease have opened up new approaches to simple, inexpensive, effective, preventive approaches. There are two parts of the oxidation problem to consider. First, we should avoid eating food that contains oxidized fats (primarily candy, cakes, pies, cookies, pastry, and other foods containing powdered milk and powdered eggs). Second, we can increase our intake of antioxidant nutrients by taking nutritional supplements.

LOGICAL ACTIONS

Because I am a licensed physician I can't make medical recommendations for people I have never seen. If a physician has advised you to get an angiogram, I can't

161

give you an opinion about whether or not to have the test. However, any cardiologist can follow the second opinion evaluation protocol published in the *Journal of the American Medical Association* by Thomas B. Grayboys (see Bibliography) and patients can request that they be evaluated in a similar way.

Possibly you may be one of the few people in whom an angiogram can be justified after the completion of tests that measure the function of the left ventricle (an isotope scan of echocardiogram). In that case I would advise trying to get a quantitative angiogram because of the accuracy problem with ordinary angiograms. Unfortunately, you will probably be unsuccessful in this effort.

I can't decide for you if cabbage surgery or a balloon job might be worthwhile. I *can* point out other courses of action that are well backed by the medical literature, ideas you may wish to consider. I can also quote the opinion of professor Braunwald of Harvard Medical School who advises against surgical procedures on the heart unless chest pains are present that persist despite efforts to relieve them.

PREVENTION OF CORONARY ARTERY DISEASE

Everyone agrees that preventing coronary artery disease is preferable to being treated after it strikes. Up to now the medical establishment has not offered preventive steps that work. Once again, you must decide what steps seem logical and feel right for you. The decision is yours more than your doctor's

I am not against reducing the intake of fat in the diet. Most Americans could stand to lose a few pounds. High fat consumption is associated with an increased rate of colon cancer and may aggravate diabetes. This is believed to occur because high fat diets generally are low in protective antioxidants. However, the lower fat diet of the American Heart Association fails to help because it does not address other dietary changes that are more important than fat intake.

FOODS TO EAT

I advise patients to eat fresh natural foods as much as possible, the same as our ancestors consumed prior to about 1850. People who lived before that time had no choice but to eat foods that had not been refined or processed. This eating pattern helped to keep them free of coronary artery disease, until they began to eat refined carbohydrates.

Vegetables should be purchased fresh, then cooked briefly in a wok or steamer, or eaten raw. If vegetables are boiled the water containing leached minerals should be consumed in the form of a soup of broth.

Avoid commercially canned or frozen vegetables. Both suffer significant losses of minerals during the washing step at the factory. In addition, canned vegetables experience a significant loss (i.e., 80 percent) of specific vitamins that are easily destroyed by heat (vitamins B-6, folic acid, vitamin C, and pantothenic acid). The first vitamins discovered, vitamins B-1, B-2, and B-3 are relatively resistant to heat damage. This finding led nutritionists to conclude that canned vegetables are a close equivalent to fresh vegetables. They continue to say this despite newer evidence to the contrary.

Fresh eggs are safe to consume as you would normally prepare them for breakfast in your own kitchen. They can be boiled, poached, scrambled, cooked into an omelet, or even fried with a little butter. The air (oxygen) exposure involved in these forms of cooking is too small to cause any significant damage. Humans have been eating eggs this way throughout the course of history.

Eggs should not be consumed as powdered eggs, or in cakes, cookies and other baked goods because of oxidative damage that results from prolonged air exposure. I advise patients to avoid low fat egg substitutes from the processed food industry. These products are less nourishing than eggs in spite of what their brand names imply. They owe their very existence to phobias attached to the cholesterol theory.[1]

We should eat grains in the form of whole grains. The first ingredient listed on a loaf of bread should read, *100 percent whole wheat flour*, not *enriched flour* or *unbleached* flour (unbleached flour is simply sifted flour that has been allowed to turn white spontaneously without the use of bleaching agents).

Other foods recommended are fresh fruits in season, as well as all other animal products in moderation. This list can include beef, fish, rabbit, chicken, turkey, pork, and wild game, as well as cheese, milk, and yogurt.

FOODS TO AVOID

Avoid refined and processed foods. A food qualifies to be called processed if it has passed through a factory. Almost all steps in which food is frozen, canned, sifted, or heated will reduce nutritional quality to some degree. Processed foods come in containers, such as bottles, cans, boxes, and packages. Processed and refined foods include ice cream, pies, cakes, TV dinners, most fast foods, refined sugar, white flour bread, and white rice.

You can't tell much about different breads by their deceptive names or appearances. Bread that is brown in color is usually made with white flour that has been dyed. The designation *wheat* bread is meaningless because *white* and *wheat* bread both come from wheat. *Crushed wheat* bread is still made with white flour as are most *seven grain* breads. We should also choose brown rice over white rice, even if it does take longer to cook.

So called *cold pressed* or *naturally pressed* oils safe to use in home made salad dressings, but not for cooking. The problem with vegetable oils is that structural changes are induced in fatty acid molecules when they are heated for many hours at high temperatures. Therefore, I recommend against using all the common brands of vegetable oil and salad dressings, as well as *all* margarines. Margarines sold in health food stores are no different.

Avoid anything that has been *hydrogenated*. Hydrogenation requires high heat treatment that changes *cis* bonds to *trans* bonds. Avoid all foods that have been deep fried. It is preferable to fry with a small amount of butter. Butter and other saturated fats are not subject to structural changes when heated because of their chemical structure (they have no double bonds).

After discussing the egg issue with patients in my office, I am amazed at the number of people who still ask if frozen liquid egg substitutes are good for them.

Weanling Rats Fed Whole Eggs Or Egg Beaters

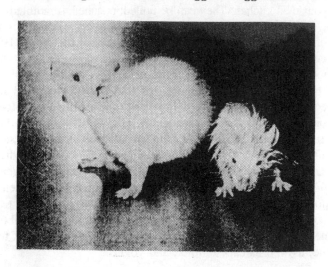

Rat pup on right is representative of the Egg Beaters group. Source: Navidi, M.K., *Pediatrics* 1974; 53:565-566. Reproduced by permission of *Pediatrics*.

This demonstrates the powerful brainwashing effects of good industry advertising. I like to respond by showing them a picture of two young rats that were participants in a feeding study.

At the beginning of the study pregnant rats were divided into two groups and were fed different foods. The same diets were continued throughout pregnancy, weaning, and in offspring after weaning. One group was fed only fresh eggs that had been frozen, then thawed. The other group ate only thawed *Egg Beaters*, one of the liquid no-cholesterol egg substitutes we have been encouraged to eat as part of the effort to reduce cholesterol in the diet.

One picture amply describes the results. The *Egg Beaters* rat pups died of malnutrition a few days after the photo was taken, about four weeks after they were weaned.

Defenders of the processed food industry would say that this study is of no importance to humans because people would never eat just one food. The common defensive phrase is: *any nutritional deficiencies will be made up from other foods.* The problem is, in the case of Americans, the other foods commonly consumed also are depleted of essential nutrients.

Be suspicious of anything that has a printed ingredient list on it. Fresh foods, such as bananas, beets, and fish, don't come with ingredient lists printed on them. Learn to trust mother nature and her natural, fresh foods, not the profit generating products of the powerful $280 billion processed food industry.

Beware of the use of the word *natural*. The word has no standardized meaning and is not regulated. Many processed foods are being advertised as being *natural*.

According to common attitudes of the processed food industry, if an ingredient in one of their products was once a natural food, the end product can be called natural as well. Therefore, we are told in advertisements that sugar and corn syrup are *natural* sweeteners because they come form cane and corn. In addition, heat treated corn oil containing harmful *trans* fatty acids is advertised as being pure.

PROTECTING THE BOTTOM LINE

Food processing companies have found that most people eat a fairly constant number of calories each day. They also are aware they can make a lot more money selling highly processed foods than fresh vegetables (i.e., potato chips compared to fresh potatoes). Therefore, the only way food manufacturers can continue to increase their profits is to manipulate consumers into eating more and more processed foods. They attempt to succeed in this effort through advertising. Therefore, to stay healthy it is wise to avoid most food products that are advertised. Nutritious fresh foods seldom are advertised.

CHEATING

Many patients tell me these guidelines are too difficult to follow. I am certainly aware of this. It is hard to be strict in following these recommendations in this modern era, though many highly motivated people do so on a daily basis. Some have learned the hard way that they have no choice but to be strict. When they cheat they become noticeably ill.

Most people will make compromises at times though it still is a good idea to follow the recommendations as much as is practical. When you break the diet for a birthday or holiday, as the average person will, it is best to get back on the *straight and narrow* as soon as possible. You might also consider swallowing a few additional antioxidant supplements (i.e., vitamin C, E, and beta-carotene) to protect you from the damage.

People also complain about the increased cost of eating fresh foods compared to other choices. This question reminds me of a television advertisement for a motor oil. A mechanic tells us that we can pay him now for an oil change, or pay him later for major engine repairs. Which is cheaper, paying 15 or 20 percent more for nourishing food now and keeping your health, or paying exorbitant medical bills in the future, suffering poor health, and possibly going through some surgical procedure?

Supermarkets respond to buying patterns of their customers. If demand for certain foods go up, the store will stock more of those items and the price will come down. They really don't have a vested interest in this subject as long as people continue to buy food from their store.

Actually, some beneficial changes have been occurring. Sales of fresh vegetables are way up and sales of canned vegetables are way down compared to 15 years ago. Sales of whole wheat bread also are up. When these buying patterns become known and accepted, food processors may see the light and find ways to produce healthy, nutritious, tasty foods.

SUPPLEMENTS

Certainly, it is best to receive our essential nutrients, vitamins, and minerals in food. Primitives did quite well and never heard of nutritional supplements. However, our food supply is not the same as it once was. Because of legitimate doubts about the nutritional content of even fresh foods, and the proven benefits of increasing the intake of antioxidants, supplementation has become a logical step.

A reasonable approach is to take a multivitamin/mineral compound that contains a long list of nutrients, then take a small number of additional products. This avoids ending up gulping handfuls of pills from scores of different bottles. In an extreme example of that practice, I once saw a little old lady who lined up 72 bottles of supplements across my desk, then asked me which ones she really needed to take.

It is possible to buy multivitamin/mineral products that contain levels close to those listed below in Table 1. It is best to find a product that divides daily doses of supplements into several pills, so one or two pills can be taken with each meal. Taking a multivitamin pill just once a day with one meal doesn't make much sense. Supplements can help in the metabolism of each meal.

TABLE 1
Approximate Total Supplement Levels Per Day

Vitamin A	5,000 to 1,000 IU
Beta-carotene	5,000 IU
Vitamin D	100 IU
Vitamin K	60 mcg
Vitamin C	1,500 mg
Vitamin B-1	100 mg
Vitamin B-2	50 mg
Vitamin B-3	200 mg
Vitamin B-5	500 mg
Vitamin B-6	25 mg
Folic Acid	800 mcg
Calcium	500 mg
Magnesium	500 mg
Copper	2 mg
Zinc	20 mg
Manganese	20 mg
Iodine	150 mcg
Chromium	200 mcg
Selenium	200 mcg
Molybdenum	100 mcg
Vanadium	25 mcg
Boron	2 mg

This list should be modified to accommodate local conditions. For example, if a person lives in a geographic area that has high selenium levels in the soil and a lot of local food is eaten, additional selenium should be avoided.

Vitamin D is listed at only 25 percent of the RDA because high doses cause experimental atherosclerosis in animals and are used in that manner.

Menstruating women need extra iron. Other people don't need iron supplements unless they are deficient in iron. An excessive amount of iron in the body has been associated with an increased risk of atherosclerosis.[2] So much for the condition of *iron poor blood.*

The calcium/magnesium ratio is 1 to 1 in this supplement list because Americans tend to be more deficient in magnesium than in calcium, despite the advertising hype from the dairy industry.

Most people will benefit from taking extra vitamin C, probably in the range of 1,000 to 3,000 mg a day. This may need to be reduced if bowel upset occurs. This level helps many people maintain bowel regularity. It is a good idea to take two or three cod liver oil capsules daily as a source of ecisopentaenoic acid (EPA).

LABORATORY TESTS

Some laboratory tests have special value in relation to coronary artery disease. A small list follows:

Lipoprotein (a)

This is probably the test with greatest predictive value for the risk of developing coronary artery disease. This test is now available from several reference laboratories.

Ferritin

A measurement of iron level in the blood. When the ferritin level is high it is wise to avoid iron supplements and reduce the intake of foods with high iron content, such as beef. It also may be a good idea to donate some blood periodically to bring the level down.

Platelet Aggregation

A measurement of the tendency of platelets to want to stick to each other. If this test is normal, then daily doses of aspirin are unnecessary and the side effects can be avoided.

Red Cell Magnesium Level

One of the tests of tissue levels of magnesium. Be certain the test is being done on a specimen of red cells. Serum levels are more easily available but much less reliable.

BEWARE OF CHOLESTEROL-LOWERING DRUGS

About all I can say here is to repeat that four large studies have shown that overall death rates go *up* with the use of cholesterol-lowering drugs, not down.

Cholesterol-lowering drugs don't lower levels of lipoprotein (a), which may turn out to be the most important blood test in determining risk of a heart attack. I would not consider using these drugs myself until someone produces evidence that the benefits of their use outweigh the risks.

WHEN PREVENTION FAILS

If I had a heart attack I would want to be transported to a coronary care unit immediately and be placed on a machine to monitor the rhythm of my heart. I would also want to receive magnesium by injection, preferably by intravenous drip as described in Chapter 8. If I couldn't talk my doctor into giving me magnesium, I would want to receive an intravenous injection of the cheaper clot dissolving drug, streptokinase. Then I would want to ride out the attack and simply recuperate without having a treadmill or angiogram.

Many cardiologists like to order angiograms about two weeks after a heart attack to see what the *road map* of the circulation of the heart looks like. There are good reasons to not go along with this. First, as the *second opinion clinic* studies have shown, if the left ventricle of the heart is pumping normally, no angiogram is indicated at all. This was the case in over 80 percent of patients with coronary artery disease. Therefore, a more useful test would be one that measures the *ejection fraction*. Second, the angiogram test proposed will undoubtedly be of the inaccurate variety.

According to Dr. Henry Braunwald, professor of medicine at Harvard Medical School, doctors should consider recommending cabbage surgery only when chest pains can't be controlled through other means. The same advice should apply to balloon procedures. If you do go ahead and have a balloon procedure, try to avoid becoming fodder for some balloon passing cardiologist who is just learning the procedure, a person referred to in the trade as a *beginning dilator*.

It is reasonable to have a treadmill test sometime after recuperating from a heart attack, as well as one of the non-invasive tests that measure the function (ejection fraction) of the left ventricle (an echocardiogram or isotope scan). Doctors can follow the evaluation methods of Marks at Duke University and Grayboys at Harvard (see references in Bibliography). The articles themselves can be found easily in the medical library of any hospital. At the present time few physicians seem to want to believe these studies exist.

After these tests, yearly death rate risk can be estimated with a high degree of accuracy. Most people will find themselves in the low risk category. For that group angiograms, cabbage surgery, and balloon jobs are not indicated. They add additional risk, suffering, and cost, but no benefits.

EDTA chelation therapy, combined with a fresh food diet, nutritional supplements, and other lifestyle changes, might be considered for anyone with coronary artery disease. Many of these alternative steps complement each other. Sometime in the future I expect to hear of malpractice suits being filed for failure to fully inform people of these choices before coercing them into surgical procedures.

If a patient survives his heart attack and still has chest pains that can't be controlled with drugs, he may be a candidate for cabbage surgery or balloon job to try to relieve the pain. But, there are other options. One is to load up on antioxidants and follow Dean Ornish's program, the program accepted by health experts as proving the disease can be reversed in a high percentage of heart patients. Ornish's program is not for everyone, but patients have a right to know about it and should be offered a choice.

If everyone followed these steps, much of the coronary artery disease problem could be prevented. In addition, the number of cabbages and balloon procedures would fall to very low levels.

ACTIONS OF POLITICAL NATURE

Politics play a large role in the direction of the management of coronary artery disease. By your actions you may help beneficial changes may occur.

Patients with heart problems should become assertive and insist that their heart status be evaluated by the methods used in the second opinion clinic studies described. This would put aggressive cabbage surgeons and *quick draw* catheter passing cardiologists on notice that they are going to be held more accountable for their actions than they have been in the past.

You can vote at the supermarket. By selecting fresh natural foods you can help insure their continued availability and a wider selection in the future. Modern transportation systems make it possible for fresh foods to be available anywhere in the country, even in the middle of winter.

I would suggest that you refrain from donating money to the American Heart Association until that organization shows signs of changing its direction. When volunteers ask you for a donation and you decline, let them know why you are not giving them money. They may not understand what you are talking about, but I am certain you will have their full attention.

If bills are reintroduced into Congress that would restrict your ability to protect your own health, get into the fight. Contact your senator and representatives and let them know your opinions. If you fail to act you may not be able to have easy access to herbs, amino acids, vitamin, and mineral supplements in the future. Access is already restricted in most European countries. Well funded and powerful vested interests would like to shut down the nutritional supplement industry in this country as well.

CONCLUSIONS

The hereditary tendency for coronary artery disease becomes apparent when humans eat poorly and follow destructive lifestyles. The history of the disease demonstrates it is preventable. Recent studies have proven it also can be reversed. Once present the disease usually can be successfully treated with approaches that remain controversial and are poorly investigated by a medical establishment that doesn't show any sign of wanting to progress.

My hope is that individuals will become aware of these findings, reclaim responsibility for their own health, and force the medical establishment to stop the current mismanagement of heart disease. It is time for the carnage to stop.

14

EPILOGUE

I wrote this book primarily for my patients. There is so much to unlearn and learn about heart disease only a small amount can be summarized during a one hour office visit. Also, it has been found that the average patient doesn't absorb much in one sitting. Most people are lucky if they remember 10 percent of what a doctor says to them during an office visit. A book format helps to get around that problem.

WHY WRITE THIS BOOK?

The overall tone of the book is highly critical of how the medical establishment handles heart disease. If medicine did a better job in preventing and treating heart disease, I would never have felt a compulsion to become involved in this subject. I did so because I am frustrated in seeing many worthless approaches proliferate, even glorified, within conventional medicine, while more effective, cheaper, and safer approaches remain dormant and unstudied on the shelf.

I also felt a public responsibility. The bypass and balloon industries remind me of drunken drivers who are veering back and forth down a highway out of control and causing a lot of mayhem. I felt a moral obligation to try to stop them before they do more harm.

I don't consider myself a be anti-doctor. I believe most physicians start out with the best of intentions to help their patients. I believe that most bypass surgeons and balloon passing cardiologists honestly believe that their pet plumbing procedures help people. But doctors are nothing more than products of the system in which they function, and they practice the way in which they have been indoctrinated. We all start out being brainwashed in medical school.

Unfortunately the system programs the little computer discs in physicians' brains as if the tracings are being imprinted in stone. Once programmed in medical school, concepts that seem foreign don't compute. Doctors assume that they have been taught the *good stuff*, that their trusted professors have sifted out treatments that don't work. Therefore, if a treatment approach is not taught in medical school it is rejected automatically. An assumption also is made that the professors have actually evaluated the methods they attack, and done so without malice or bias. This is almost never the case.

170

Students are not selected for admission to medical schools on the basis of demonstrating an ability to think independently, creatively, or even logically. Most are science majors who have a high aptitude for memorizing tons of meaningless minutia and regurgitating the stuff on tests. Therefore, if patient after patient tells a doctor of improvements they experienced after using some simple, safe, alternative medicine approach, it makes no impression. They might as well try spitting into the wind, or asking the doctor to change religions. In the business of modern medicine beliefs rule the day while facts frequently are rejected or ignored.

THE ENIGMA OF CHRONIC DISEASES

Medicine has made great advances in the past 100 years in many areas. The major contagious diseases in children are under control. Congenital defects, infections and other acute medical problems usually are handled well with the methods of modern medicine. I believe in treating strep throat with penicillin, removing the appendix when it is inflamed, and injecting children with the non-contagious, killed form of polio vaccine (so as to avoid infecting other people as is used in Scandinavia).

However, medicine fails when it attempts to treat chronic degenerative diseases with the same approaches it uses successfully in acute medical problems. This is a major problem because of all modern maladies that are brought to the attention of doctors, 80 percent are chronic.

Lacking any basic understanding of what may be causing diseases of physical degeneration, treatments generally involve the prescription of some symptoms suppressing synthetic petroleum product. Medicine has entered a new era of aggression in which the body is viewed as being a fancy machine. Damaged parts can be replaced as if your body was an old car (i.e., replacement of kidneys, eye lenses, hip joints, hearts, lungs, livers, intestines). This may not sound compassionate, but we could get a lot more bang for the buck using these health care dollars providing adequate nutrition to pregnant women in impoverished ghettos.

Most modern drugs work by blocking enzymes in our cells that carry out normal chemical processes. Many are even called *blockers*, such as calcium channel blockers, beta blockers, and histamine blockers. Other drugs have the word *anti* in front of them, such as antihistamines and antispasmodics. Is it any wonder that modern drugs are rife with side effects?

Eli Lilly, founder of the drug company that bears his name, is remembered for a famous quote: "A drug with no side effects is no drug at all." It should be no surprise that medical treatment is the seventh leading cause of death in the United States, and that death rates fall when doctors go on strike.

For many drugs the mechanism of action remains totally unknown. The majority of drugs smother symptoms of the problem and make patients feel better. Most drugs are developed in a hit or miss manner and generally don't have anything to do with causes of a disease. The basic problem continues to smolder along unchanged.

THE QUICK FIX SYNDROME

This problem continues on almost unnoticed by a public that has been conditioned to believe a *quick fix* exists for every problem. In the *Physician's Desk Reference* (a book in which drug companies pay to list drugs they are currently pushing) symptoms are listed alphabetically with drugs itemized under every symptom. This makes it easy for a doctor to prescribe a drug about which he knows nothing. When in doubt, look up a symptom and prescribe. It also makes it easy for impostors to pass themselves off as physicians.

In one well publicized case an impostor hung out his shingle as Doctor X, M.D. After asking each patient about his or her current problem, he would excuse himself to "do something in the next room." He would go back to his office, look up the symptom in the *Physician's Desk Reference*, pick a drug at random and write out a prescription.

What impressed me was that this fellow, whose only medical experience was gained while working in a hospital as a janitor, developed a successful practice and a devoted clientele. In other words, he did as well in his practice as *real* doctors who had been to medical school. Some of his patients thought he walked on water, though he had never set foot inside a medical school, the usual requirement.

Another recent impostor rose to an academic position in a west coast medical school. He even served as editor of a popular textbook in pediatrics and was a respected member of his department. This shows how medicine can be practiced *by the book* as long as a prescription pad is handy.

In other areas we have been conditioned to connect problems with quick fixes as if we are playing a one word association game. For osteoporosis we think of calcium. For tooth decay we think of sugar and fluoride. For heart disease we think of cholesterol and cabbages. For bugs under the sink we think of *Raid*. All of these are complex problems, yet we react and simplify according to our conditioning.

RESEARCH TOWERS OF BABEL

In a general state of confusion, research efforts have been launched individually against each disease of physical degeneration. Each malady ends up with a separate fund-raising effort, bureaucracy, and research headquarters building. We have separate buildings and organizations for cancer, diabetes, stroke, arthritis, heart disease, and a long list of other maladies, some quite obscure. All compete for donations and research dollars. Medical specialists divide up the body in a similar manner. No effort is made to look for common threads that tie degenerative diseases together. Connections are subtle, but they are there.

When it comes to coronary artery disease, treatments would be almost laughable if many were not so risky, costly, traumatic, and ineffective. Treatment decisions usually are made on the basis of inaccurate angiograms. Ignored are published second opinion studies which have used commonly available non-invasive tests to determine left ventricular function. The function of the heart is to pump blood. Its efficiency as a pump is what is critical to the body, not some so-called *road map* on an inaccurate angiogram.

Hopefully efforts at cost containment in medicine will lead to mandatory second opinion evaluations before surgical procedures on the heart can be done (or paid for by insurance). If methods described were implemented before most angiograms were done, this would almost close off the tunnel through which people pass on their way to cabbages and balloon jobs.

Billions of health care dollars could be saved and patients would do just as well if cabbage surgeons and invasive cardiologists were disarmed. The government could even extend a helping hand and offer to retrain bypass surgeons, at least the minuscule number who haven't made their millions yet. It would make good sense to force them to shift their efforts into more useful pursuits. They have been behaving like plumbers for many years now. Let them become *real* plumber.

PEOPLE IN THE FUTURE WILL SAY "SHAME ON US"

We regard medical treatments of 100 years ago as being unscientific and barbaric. I have no doubt that 100 years from now people will make similar comments about medicine as practiced now, especially in regard to cabbage surgery and cancer treatments. Even now, medicines' major treatments are commonly referred to as cutting, burning, and poisoning. People of the future will wonder why we did not begin to prevent degenerative diseases with the knowledge we now possess. They will also wonder why we used surgical procedures so frequently in the treatment of coronary artery disease.

MEDICAL WITCH HUNTS

Many people cautioned me not to put this book into print. If I was a younger physician I would never have considered doing anything so flamboyant and dangerous. Establishment medicine does not welcome criticism, either from outside or from within. Frequently the establishment lashes out at physicians who have ventured outside the wall of dogma of the *Church of Modern Medicine.*

Many of my colleagues in *alternative medicine* have been dragged before state disciplinary boards for doing nothing more than practicing a different form of medicine than the average physician. In one case a patient had begun chemotherapy but stopped after one treatment because of severe side effects. After being successfully treated with alternative approaches the man returned to his cancer specialist (oncologist) for a check up to see how he was doing. The cancer (a lymphoma) was gone.

The cancer specialist became upset about this invasion of his turf. He wrote a letter to the state disciplinary board complaining about the treating doctor and her unorthodox methods. After a lengthy legal battle the board took away the physician's license to practice.

Apparently, it does not pay to be a highly effective alternative practitioner. The more *effective* the unorthodox healer, the more threatened the medical establishment becomes. The more threatened it feels, the more viciously it will lash out against a *wayward* doctor.

It is ironic that in the United States we have more personal freedoms than in most countries in the world, yet we have the most restrictive medical system. In contrast, in the People's Republic of China, physicians are allowed the greatest freedom of choice in the methods they might use.

The most logical approach medicine could take would be to treat people with the most effective, safest, approaches to their problems, regardless of the origin of the methods, and without prejudice. Unfortunately, inertia, biases, and profit motives get in the way.

You need to be informed that there may be options in treating a problem, not just the narrow road leading to drugs or surgery. However, you will need to educate yourself in this area because few physicians know about other options and therefore none will be offered. Only by being informed of all of your options can a truly *informed consent* be granted for a procedure.

I close now with best wishes to everyone. I hope you will benefit from reading this book.

BIBLIOGRAPHY

REFERENCES FOR YOUR DOCTOR

This book was written for ordinary people, not physicians. I have been highly critical of many ways that conventional medicine handles coronary artery disease. However, I did not dream up the criticism out of the clear blue sky. All I have done is read the recent medical literature and translate it for you.

The most important studies on which I have based my conclusions have appeared in a small number of prominent medical journals. These publications are in wide circulation and available in the medical library of most hospitals. Many physicians also subscribe to these same journals.

There are several things that you might do with this information. First, you can go to a nearby hospital and read the small number of articles I have listed below. Most hospital medical libraries are open to the public and medical librarians are usually friendly to those with serious intent. Visitors are generally allowed to read on the premises.

Even though you may not be able to decipher the medical jargon in the body of most articles the summaries are usually written more clearly. You also can encourage your doctor to read the articles on this list by photocopying them and presenting them to him or her as a gift!

SOME ARTICLES SHOWING THE ORDINARY ANGIOGRAM TO BE INACCURATE

1. Zir, L.M., et al, Interobserver Variability in Coronary Angiography, *Circulation* 1976; 53:627-632. A study in which four experts at Massachusetts General Hospital independently interpreted the same areas of blockage on the same high quality angiograms. Interpretations of blockages in coronary arteries varied by as much as 100 percent.

2. Grodin, C.M., et al, Discrepancies Between Cineangiographic (Angiogram) and Postmortem (Autopsy) Findings in Patients with Coronary Artery Disease and Recent Myocardial Revascularization (Bypass Surgery), *Circulation* 1974; 49:703-708. This study compared X-ray readings of angiograms with the actual arteries of people who died soon after a cabbage surgery. Correlation was poor.

3. Arnett, E.N., et al, Coronary Artery Narrowing in Coronary Heart Disease: Comparison of Cineangiographic (Angiogram) and Necropsy (Autopsy) Findings, *Annals of Internal Medicine* 1979; 91:350-356. This study also compared X-ray readings of angiograms with actual arteries of people who died soon after a cabbage surgery.

4. White, Carl W., et al, Does Visual Interpretation of the Coronary Arteriogram Predict the Physiologic Importance of a Coronary Stenosis? *New England Journal of Medicine* 1984; 310:819-824. This study compared ordinary angiogram readings with doppler ultrasound measurements taken directly on arteries with the chest open during heart surgery. The doppler readings were accepted as being 100 percent accurate. No correlation was found between the two methods. The authors cautioned against using information from ordinary angiograms as the basis for doing surgical procedures.

5. Angiographic Misreading and Conflicts Found Rife, *Medical World News*, December 24, 1979. Unpublished study presented at an American Heart Association meeting. The same angiograms were read in three institutions. A few weeks later the same angiograms were recirculated and read by the same experts. Widespread discrepancies were found even among readings by the same person on two different dates.

MAJOR ARTICLES SHOWING THAT PEOPLE WHO RECEIVE CORONARY ARTERY BYPASS SURGERY DON'T LIVE ANY LONGER THAN THOSE TREATED MEDICALLY

1. Eleven Year Survival in the Veterans Administration Randomized Trial of Coronary Bypass Surgery for Stable Angina, The Veterans Administration Coronary Artery Bypass Surgery Cooperative Study Group, *New England Journal of Medicine* 1977; 311:1333-1339. An 11-year study in 13 veterans hospitals that found the same survival rates with bypass surgery as with medical management.

2. Alderman, E.L., et al, Ten-Year Follow-up of Survival and Myocardial Infarction in the Randomized Coronary Artery Surgery Study, *Circulation* 1990; 82:1629-1646. A study of the results of bypass surgery in the hands of *better* surgeons. Results were similar to those of the Veterans Study. One highly useful finding was the patients with normal function of the left ventricle did better if managed medically, and they constituted 82 percent of the total group.

3. European Coronary Artery Surgery Study Group, Long-Term Results of a Prospective Randomized Study of Coronary Artery Bypass Surgery in Stable Angina Pectoris, *Lancet* 1982; Nov. 27, pp 1173-1180. This study found a slightly better survival rate in bypass surgery patients, but the difference was not statistically significant.

MAJOR ARTICLES SHOWING THAT PEOPLE LIVE LONGER WITH CORONARY ARTERY BYPASS SURGERY
None.

AN ARTICLE ON FOLLOW-UP OF PATIENTS WHO REFUSED CORONARY ARTERY BYPASS SURGERY

1. Hueb, W., et al, *American Journal of Cardiology* 1989; 63:155-159. One hundred fifty patients who had been advised to have coronary bypass surgery refused the operation. They were managed medically and followed for two to eight years. Annual mortality rate was 0 percent in patients with disease in one or two coronary arteries, and 1.3 percent in patients with disease in all three coronary arteries. Estimated overall probability of survival at eight years was 89 percent. In other words, these people did just fine without the surgery.

ARTICLES ON CHOLESTEROL SCREENING AND LIPID LOWERING EFFORTS

1. Hulley, Stephen, et al, Childhood Cholesterol Screening: Contraindicated, *Journal of the American Medical Association* 1992; 267:100-102. Contains the results from several studies that showed that *overall* death rates actually go up when efforts are made to lower blood cholesterols with diets or drugs.

2. Hulley, Stephen, et al, Health Policy on Blood Cholesterol, Time to Change Directions, *Circulation* 1992; 86:1026-1029. An editorial in the journal published by the American Heart Association advising a massive reduction in cholesterol screening efforts. Points out that elevated blood cholesterol is of no predicative value in children, women at any age, or men "who do not yet have manifestations of coronary artery disease (or other reasons for being at a comparable very high risk of coronary heart disease death)."

ARTICLES IN WHICH NON-INVASIVE METHODS WERE USED TO SHOW THAT MOST INVASIVE (SURGICAL) HEART PROCEDURES ARE UNNECESSARY

1. Grayboys, Thomas B., Results of a Second-Opinion Program for Coronary Artery Bypass Graft Surgery, *Journal of the American Medical Association* 1987; 258:1611-1614. Eighty-eight people were evaluated who had been seen elsewhere and advised to have cabbage surgery. After non-invasive testing bypass surgery was felt to *not* be indicated in 84 percent. Of those who followed the advice none died in the next two years.

2. Grayboys, Thomas B., et al, Results of a Second Opinion Angiography, *Journal of the American Medical Association* 1992; 268:2537-2540. One hundred sixty-eight people were evaluated who had been advised by other doctors to have angiograms. Eighty percent were found to be excellent candidates for medical management and to not need the test. During the next four years the death rate for all 168 people was only 1.1 percent per year.

3. Marks, D.B. et al, *New England Journal of Medicine* 1991; 325:849-853. Marks evaluated 613 people with suspected coronary artery disease with treadmill testing alone. A prognostic scoring system was devised and patients were categorized into high and low risk groups. Two-thirds fell into the low risk category.

Among those people the death rate was only 0.25 percent per year during the next four years.

THE BEST DOCUMENTED EVIDENCE OF REVERSAL OF OBSTRUCTIONS IN CORONARY ARTERIES

1. Ornish, Dean, et al, Can Lifestyle Changes Reverse Coronary Heart Disease? *Lancet* 1990; 336:129-133. Ornish's patients received quantitative angiograms before and after one year of an intensive diet and lifestyle program. Eighty-five percent of the people in his test group improved. The worst obstructions opened up an average of 8.6 percent in diameter during the year. The control group was placed on the American Heart Association diet. Their obstructions worsened by 4.4 percent during the year and their symptoms also worsened.

TREATMENT OF HEART ATTACK PATIENTS WITH INTRAVENOUS MAGNESIUM

1. Horner, S.M., *Circulation* 1992; 86:774-779. A combination study of 930 people admitted to hospitals with heart attacks. The intravenous administration of magnesium was associated with a 49 percent reduction in ventricular tachycardia and fibrillation. The incidence of cardiac arrest was reduced by 58 percent. Overall there was a 54 percent reduction in deaths with the use of magnesium.

A REVIEW ARTICLE ON THE OXIDATION THEORY OF ATHEROSCLEROSIS

1. Steinberg, Daniel, et al, Beyond Cholesterol, *New England Journal of Medicine* 1989; 320:915-923.

THE FIRST DESCRIPTION OF THE NEW METHOD OF QUANTITATIVE ANGIOGRAPHY

1. Brown, B.G., Quantitative Coronary Arteriography, Estimation of Dimensions, Hemodynamic Resistance, and Atheroma Mass of Coronary Artery Lesions Using the Arteriogram and Digital Computation, *Circulation* 1977; 55:329-337. This study described taking angiogram pictures from two different angles simultaneously with two X-ray cameras. The catheter was used as a scaling device. Information was analyzed by a computer. The method measures diameters of coronary arteries accurately with a range of error of 150 microns (about 1 percent error).

SUGGESTED READING

1. Carter, James, *Racketeering in Medicine: The Suppression of Alternatives*, Norfolk, VA, Hampton Roads Pub. 1992.

2. Cleave, T.L., *The Saccharine Disease*, New Canaan, CT, Keats Pub. 1974

3. Cranton, Elmer, *Bypassing Bypass*, Trout Dale, VA, Medex Pub. 1990.

4. Hall, Russ Hume, *Food For Nought*, New York, Vintage 194, 1989.

5. Moore, Thomas, *Heart Failure*, New York, Touchstone, 1989.

6. Ornish, Dean, *Dr. Dean Ornish's Program for Reversing Heart Disease*, New York, Random House 1990.

7. Whitaker, Julian M., *Reversing Heart Disease*, New York, Warner Books 1985.

8. Williams, Roger J., *Nutrition Against Disease*, New York, Bantam 1971.

REFERENCES

CHAPTER 1: MEDICAL MANAGEMENT OF CORONARY ARTERY DISEASE

1. *Medical Tribune*, April 23, 1992, p4.
2. Groin, C.M., *Circulation* 1974; 49:703.
3. Zir, L.M., et al, *Circulation* 1976: 53:627-632.
4. *Medical World News*, Dec. 24, 1979, p6.
5. White, C.W., et al, *New England Journal of Medicine* 1984; 310:819-824.
6. Brown, B.G., et al, *Circulation* 1977; 55:329-337.
7. Buchwald, H., et al, *Journal of the American Medical Association* 1992; 268:1429-1433.
8. Blankenhorn, D.H., *Controlled Clinical Trials* 1987; 8:354-387.

CHAPTER 2: OF CABBAGES AND THEIR KINGS

1. Cobb, L.A., et al, *New England Journal of Medicine* 1959; 260:1115-1118.
2. The Veterans Study, *New England Journal of Medicine* 1977; 311:1311-1339.
3. Braunwald, E., *New England Journal of Medicine* 1977; 297:661-663.
4. Alderman, E.L., et al, *Circulation* 1990; 82:1629-1646.
5. Rogers, J.J., et al, *Circulation* 1990; 82:1647-1658.
6. European Coronary Artery Surgery Study Group, *Lancet* 1982; Sept. 27. pp1173-1180.
7. Braunwald, E., *New England Journal of Medicine* 1983; 309:1181-1184.
8. McIntosh, H.D., et al, *Circulation* 1978; 57:405-431.
9. Williams, S.V., et al, *Journal of the American Medical Association* 1991; 266:810-815.
10. Moore, Thomas, *Heart Failure*, New York, Touchstone, 1989.
11. Torkel, A., *Scandanavia Journal of Thoracic and Cardiovascular Surgery*, Supplement 15, 1974.
12. Preston, T., *MD* Feb. 1985, pp104-114.
13. Winslow, C.M., *Journal of the American Medical Association* 988; 260:505-509.
14. Guerci, A.D., et al, *New England Journal of Medicine* 1989; 320:663-665.
15. Wenneker, M.B. *Journal of the American Medical Association* 1990; 264:1255-1260.

16. Goldberg, K.C., *Journal of the American Medical Association* 1992; 267:1473-1477.

17. *Wall Street Journal*, December 11, 1992.

18. Grayboys, T.B., *Journal of the American Medical Association* 1987; 258:1611-1614.

19. Marks, D.B., *New England Journal of Medicine*.

20. Hueb, W., et al, *American Journal of Cardiology* 1989; 63:155-159.

CHAPTER 3: A BALLOON IN YOUR FUTURE?

1. National Center for Health Statistics and the Commission of Professional Hospital Activities, Washington, D.C.; 1992.

2. Hartzler, G.O. *Cardiology* 1988; 5:3.

3. Grayboys, T.B., *Journal of the American Medical Association* 1989; 261:2116-2117.

4. Grayboys, T.B., *Journal of the American Medical Association* 1992; 268:2537-2540.

CHAPTER 4: WHO BENEFITS FROM CABBAGE AND BALLOON PROCEDURES?

1. Sturm, A.C., *Modern Health Care*, Sept. 23, 1988.

2. Consumer Reports, July 1992, pp446-447.

CHAPTER 5: CHOLESTEROL-PHOBIA

1. Parry, C.H., as quoted in *A Bibliography of Internal Medicine, Selected Diseases*, Arthur Bloomfield, University of Chicago Press, 1960.

2. Levine, Samuel, *Clinical Heart Disease*, Philadelphia, W.B. Saunders Co., 1950.

3. White, Paul D., *Prog Cardiovascular Dis* 1971; 14:249.

4. Table adapted from Mann, G.V., *New England Journal of Medicine* 1975; 49:1585-1590, and Levenstein, J.H. , *South African Medical Journal* 1975; 49:1585-1590.

5. *Statistical Abstracts of the United States*, United States Department of Commerce.

6. Kannel, W.B., *Journal of the American Medical Association* 1982; 247:877-880.

7. *Virchow's Archives* 1934; 249:73.

8. Nichols, A.B., *Journal of the American Medical Association* 1976; 236:1948-1953.

9. *Medical World News* June 7, 1982.

10. MRFIT death rates as quoted in Moore, Thomas, *Heart Failure*, New York, Touchstone 1989.

11. Lipids Research Clinics Program, *Journal of the American Medical Association* 1984; 251:351-364.

12. Moore, Thomas, *Heart Failure*, New York, Touchstone 1989.

13. Ibid

14. Ahrens, E.H., *Lancet* May 11, 1985, pp1085-1087.

15. Cleave, T.L., *The Saccharine Disease*, Keats Pub. New Canaan, CT 1974.

16. Biss, K., et al, *New England Journal of Medicine* 1971; 284:694-699.

17. Walker, A.R.P., et al, *British Medical Journal* 1978; 1:1336-1338.

18. Leaf, A., *Youth in Old Age*, New York, McGraw Hill 1975.

19. Benet, Sula, *How to Live to be 100*, New York, Dial Press 1976.

20. Drury, R.A., *Tropical and Geographic Medicine* 1976; 24:385-392.

21. Smith, et al, *Tropical Medicine and Hygiene* 1976; 25 (4):637-643.

22. Gsel, D., et al, *American Journal of Clinical Nutrition* 1962; 10:471.

23. Cohen, J.C., et al, *Lancet* 1962; 2:1399.

24. Lowenstein, F.W., *American Journal of Clinical Nutrition* 1964; 15:175.

25. Biss, K., et al, *New England Journal of Medicine* 1971; 284:694-699.

26. Stamler, J., et al, *Journal of the American Medical Association* 1986; 256:2823-2827.

27. Taylor, W.C., *Annals of Internal Medicine* 1987; 106:605-614.

28. Williams, R.R., et al, *Journal of the American Medical Association* 1986; 255:219-224.

29. Blankenhorn, D., et al, *Journal of the American Medical Association* 1987; 257:3233-3240.

30. Brown, Gregg, et al, *New England Journal of Medicine* 1990; 323:1289-1298.

31. Hulley, Stephen, et al, *Journal of the American Medical Association* 1992; 267:100-102.

32. Olson, R.F., *Journal of the American Medical Association* 1986; 255:2204-2207.

33. Kaunitz, H., *Journal of the American Oil Chemists Society*, Aug. 1975.

34. Mann, George, *New England Journal of Medicine* 1977; 297:664-650.

35. Mann, George, *American Heart Journal* 1978; 96:569-571.

36. Brisson, G.J., *Lipids in Human Nutrition*, Englewood NJ, Jack K. Burgess 1981.

37. Hacobs, D., et al, *Circulation* 1992; 86:1046-1060.

38. Hulley, Stephen, *Circulation* 1992; 86:1026-1029.

39. Ravnskov, U., *British Medical Journal* 1992; 305:15-19.

CHAPTER 6: WINNERS AND LOSERS FROM THE CHOLESTEROL THEORY

1. Smith, Russell, *The Cholesterol Conspiracy*, St. Louis, Warren H. Green 1991.

CHAPTER 7: METHODS THAT REALLY HELP

1. Trowell, Hugh C., *Executive Health*, Nov. 1977.

2. Price, Weston, *Nutrition and Physical Degeneration*, New Canaan, CT, Keats Pub, 1945.

3. Cleave, T.L., *The Saccharine Disease*, New Canaan, CT, Keats Pub, 1974.

4. Schaefer, Otto, *Nutrition Today*, 1971; Nov-Dec. pp8-16.

5. Cleave, T.L., *The Saccharine Disease*, New Canaan, CT, Keats Pub, 1974.

6. *Medical World News* Aug. 12, 1985.

7. Ornish, Dean, et al, *Lancet* 1990; 336:129-133.

8. Ornish, Dean, *Dr. Dean Ornish's Program for Reversing Heart Disease*, New York, Random House 1990.

9. Blankenhorn, D., et al, *Journal of the American Medical Association* 1987; 257:3233-3240.

10. Brown, Greg, *New England Journal of Medicine* 1990; 323:1289-1298.

11. Personal communication

12. Kitchell, J.R., et al, *American Journal of Cardiology* 1963; 95-100.

13. Brecher, Arlene, et al, *Forty Something Forever*, Herndon VA, Healthsavers Press 1992.

14. Olszewer, Efriam, et al, *Journal of the National Medical Association* 1990; 82:173-177.

15. Casdorph, H.R., *Journal of Advancement in Medicine* 1989; 2:131-153.

16. Casdorph, H.R., *Journal of Advancement in Medicine* 1989; 2:167-182.

17. Casdorph, H.R., *Journal of Advancement in Medicine* 1989; 2:121-129.

18. McGillem, J.J., New *England Journal of Medicine* 1988; 318:1618-1619.

19. Dudrick, Stanley J., *Annals of Surgery* 1987; 206:296-315.

20 Pottenger, Francis, *American Journal of Orthodontics and Oral Surgery* 1946; 32:467-485.

21. Steinman, Ralph R., *Journal of Dental Research* 1958; 37 #5 pp874-879.

CHAPTER 8: NUTRIENT CONNECTIONS

1. Williams, Roger, *Nutrition Against Disease*, New York, Bantam 1971.

2. Greenberg, L.D. *Proceedings of the Society for Experimental Biology and Medicine* 1951; 76:580.

3. *Bulletin of Sinai Hospital*, Detroit 1975; 23:81.

4. Williams, Roger, *The Wonderful World Within You*, New York, Bantam 1971.

5. Volkov, N.F., *Fed Proc Trans Supp* 1963; 22:T895.

6. Wacker, W.E.C., et al, *New England Journal of Medicine* 1950; 355:499.

7. Henzel, J.H., et al, in Pories, J.J., *Clinical Applications of Zinc Metabolism*, Springfield, IL, Charles Thomas Pub. 1974.

8. Roe, Daphne, *Drug Induced Nutritional Deficiencies*, Westport, CT, Avi Books 1976.

9. Crawford, T., et al, *Lancet* 1967; 1:229.

10. Anderson, T.W., *Canadian Medical Journal* 1975; 113:199-203.

11. Altura, Burton M., *Medical Tribune* Aug. 20, 1980, p3.

12. Smith, L.F., et al, *International Journal of Cardiology* 1986; 12:175-180.

13. Rasmussen, H. Sandvod, et al, *Lancet* 1986; Feb 1, pp234-236.

14. Parsons, R.S., et al, *Medical Proceedings* 1959; 5:487.

15. Horner, S.M., *Circulation* 1992; 86:774-779.

16. *Medical Tribune* Aug. 27, 1986.

17. Carroll, Harvey F., *Medical World News*, May 26, 1986.

18. Gey, K. Fred, et al, *American Journal of Clinical Nutrition* 1991; 53:326S-34S

19. Gaziano, J. Michael, *Circulation* 1990; 82-III:201

20. Gaby, A.G., *American Journal of Holistic Medicine* 1983; 5:107-120.

21. Enstrom, J.E., et al, *Epidemiology* 1992; 3:194-202.

22. Frei, Balz, *American Journal of Clinical Nutrition* 1991; 54:1113S-18S.

23. Morrison, Lester M., *Journal of the American Medical Association* 1960; 173:884-887.
24. Gaby, A.G., *Journal of Holistic Medicine* 1983; 5:107-127.
25. Shamberger, R.J., *Federation Proceedings* 1976; 35:578 abstract #3016.
26. Collipp, P.J., *New England Journal of Medicine* 1981; 302:1304.
27. Kromhout, D., *New England Journal of Medicine* 1985; 312:1206-1209.
28. Brisson, G., *Lipids in Human Nutrition*, Englewood, NJ, Jack K. Burgess 1981.
29. Kummerow, F.A., *Federation Proceedings* 1975; 33:235.
30. Kritchevsky, D., et al, *Journal of Atherosclerosis Research* 1967; 7:643.
31. Heimlich, Jane, *What Your Doctor Won't Tell You*, New York, Perennial 1990.
32. Mensink, R.P., et al, *New England Journal of Medicine* 1990; 323:439-445.
33. Rose, G.A., *British Medical Journal* 1965; 1:1531.
34. Cleave, T.L., *The Saccharine Disease*, New Canaan CT, Keats Pub. 1974.
35. Hunt, A.D.J., et al, *Pediatrics* 1954; 13:140.
36. Werbach, M.R., *Nutritional Influences on Illness*, Tarzana CA, Third Line Press, Inc. 1987.

CHAPTER 9: PREVENT ARTERIAL "RUST"

1. Steinberg, D., et al, *New England Journal of Medicine* 1989; 320:915-923.
2. Cathcart, M.K., et al, *Journal of Leukocyte Biology* 1985; 38:341-350.
3. Tolonen, M., et al, *Biologic and Trace Element Research* 1988; pp221-228.
4. Salonen, J.T., et al, *American Journal of Clinical Nutrition* 1991; 53(5) p1222-1229
5. Boorman, G.A., et al, *Toxicol Pathol* 1987; 15(4) p451-456.
6. Petty, M.A. et al, *European Journal of Pharmacology* 1990; 180(1):119-127.
7. Rath, M., et al, *Arteriosclerosis* 1989; 8:579-592.
8. Rader, D.J., et al, *Journal of the American Medical Association* 1992; 267:1109-1111.

CHAPTER 10: OTHER RISK FACTORS

1. Faris, J.V., et al, *American Journal of Cardiology* 1976; 37:617-622.
2. Soloman, Henry, *The Exercise Myth*, New York, Harcourt Brace and Jovanovich 1984.
3. Anderson, R.A., et al, *American Journal of Clinical Nutrition* 1982; 35:840
4. Douglass, John M., *Annals of Internal Medicine* 1975; 82:61-62.
5. Henry, J.P., et al, *Stress, Health, and the Social Environment*, New York, Springer-Verlag 1977.
6. Yudkin, J., *Sweet and Dangerous*, New York, Bantam, 1972.
7. *Associated Press*, July 2, 1992.

CHAPTER 11: TRYING TO UNDERSTAND
CORONARY ARTERY DISEASE

1. Hurley, L., *The Johns Hopkins Medical Journal* 1981; 148:1-10.
2. Smithells, R.W., *Lancet* 1980; I:399-340.

3. Smithells, R.W., *Archives of Diseases of Children* 1981; 56:911-918.
4. Holmes, L.B., *Journal of the American Medical Association* 1988; 260:31.
5. *Medical Tribune*, October 22, 1992.

CHAPTER 12: BIASES AND POLITICS
1. Davies, N.E., et al, *Journal of the American Medical Association* 1983; 249:912-915.
2. Herbert, V., *Journal of the American Medical Association* 1974; 230:241-242.
3. Newmark, H.L., *American Journal of Clinical Nutrition* 1976; 29:645-649.
4. Personal communication
5. Nightingale, S., *Journal of the American Medical Association* 1992; 268:1828.
6. Personal communication
7. Brecher, A., et al, *Forty Something Forever*, Herndon VA, Healthsavers Press 1992.
8. Smith, R.L., *The Cholesterol Conspiracy*, St. Louis, Warren H. Green Pub. 1991.
9. *Townsend Letter for Doctors*, Jan. 1992, pp63-64.
10. Sloth-Nielson, J., et al, *American Journal of Surgery* 1991; 142:122-125.
11. Frackelton, J.P., *Townsend Newsletter for Doctors*, July 1992.
12. Brodeur, Paul, *The Zapping of America*, Wade Rawson 1977.

CHAPTER 13: REASONABLE ACTIONS
1. Navidi, M.K., et al, *Pediatrics* 1974; 53:565-566.
2. Salonen, J., et al, *Circulation* 1992; 86(3):803-811.

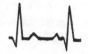

ABOUT THE AUTHOR

Charles T. McGee has an unusual background for a physician. After completion of specialty training in obstetrics and gynecology he treated primitive lifestyle Indians in the Andes mountains of Ecuador for one year in a land based Project HOPE program. He had a chance to see first hand the commonly observed pattern that primitive lifestyle people did not suffer from heart attacks, high blood pressure, strokes, diabetes, and a long list of other disease that are common in more developed countries.

Following this he served in the United States Public Health Service for two years as an Epidemic Intelligence Officer at the Centers for Disease Control (CDC). This involved becoming aware of the fields of biostatistics and epidemiology.

In 1974 he began to study traditional Chinese medicine. That led to investigations into nutrition, ecologic issues, and other alternative medical therapies from around the world. He discovered that conventional medicine discriminated against many treatment approaches that had value. He gradually modified his practice to concentrate on chronic diseases that are handled poorly by orthodox medicine.

In 1987 Dr. McGee began a series of trips to China, serving as a consultant to several innovative medical programs. In Hainan Province he again had the opportunity to observe a large group of people who remain almost totally free of diseases of physical degeneration (and heart attacks) and probably have the best health pattern in the world, living to an average age of 87.

Dr. McGee is also the author of three additional books *How to Survive Modern Technology*, *Miracle Healing From China...Qigong*, and *Healing Energies*.

INDEX

187

THE HEALING MIRACLES OF COCONUT OIL

If there was an oil you could use for your daily cooking needs that helped protect you from heart disease, cancer, and other degenerative conditions, improved your digestion, strengthened your immune system, and helped you lose excess weight, would you be interested?

No such oil exists you say? Not so! There is an oil that can do all this and more. No, it's not olive oil, it's not canola oil, or safflower oil or any of the oils commonly used for culinary purposes. It's not flaxseed oil, evening primrose oil, or any of the oils sold as dietary supplements. It's not rare or exotic. It's ordinary coconut oil.

But, isn't coconut oil a saturated fat? And isn't saturated fat bad? Because coconut oil is primarily a saturated oil, it has been blindly labeled as bad. It is lumped right along with beef tallow and lard with the assumption that they all carry the same health risks. However, researchers have clearly shown that fat from coconuts, a plant source, acts differently than the saturated fat from animal sources. The oil from the coconut is unique in nature and provides many health benefits obtainable from no other source.

What Coconut Oil *Does Not* Do:
• Does not contribute to atherosclerosis or heart disease
• Does not promote platelet stickiness which leads to blood clot formation
• Does not contain cholesterol
• Does not increase blood cholesterol
• Does not promote cancer or any other degenerate disease
• Does not contribute to weight problems

What Coconut Oil *Does* Do:
• Reduces risk of atherosclerosis and related illnesses
• Reduces risk of cancer and other degenerative conditions
• Helps prevent bacterial, viral, and fungal (including yeast) infections
• Supports immune system function
• Helps prevent osteoporosis
• Helps control diabetes
• Promotes weight loss
• Supports healthy metabolic function
• Provides an immediate source of energy
• Supplies fewer calories than other fats
• Supplies important nutrients necessary for good health
• Improves digestion and nutrient absorption
• Has a mild delicate flavor
• Is highly resistant to spoilage (long shelf life)
• Is heat resistant (the healthiest oil for cooking)
• Helps keep skin soft and smooth
• Helps prevent premature aging and wrinkling of the skin
• Helps protect against skin cancer and other blemishes

Coconut oil has been called *the healthiest dietary oil on earth*. If you're not using coconut oil for your daily cooking and body care needs you're missing out on one of nature's most amazing health products. The health benefits of coconut oil are clearly explained and documented in the book *The Healing Miracles of Coconut Oil* by Bruce Fife, N.D.

Look for this book in your local bookstore or health food store. If it is not available in your area you can order it directly from the publisher. To order *The Healing Miracles of Coconut Oil* send $18.00 (post paid) to HealthWise Publications, P.O. Box 25203, Colorado Springs, CO 80936.